Food Allergies:
A Recipe For Success At School

Food Allergies:
A Recipe For Success At School

Information, Recommendations and Inspiration
for Families and School Personnel

JAN HANSON, M.A.

authorHOUSE®

AuthorHouse™
1663 Liberty Drive
Bloomington, IN 47403
www.authorhouse.com
Phone: 1-800-839-8640

This publication is intended to provide information in regard to the subject matter covered, but does not provide legal or medical advice. Any application of recommendations offered in this book is at the reader's discretion. The author and the publisher specifically disclaim any and all liability arising directly or indirectly from the use or application of any information contained in this book. If legal or medical advice is required, the services of a competent medical or legal professional should be sought.

Published by AuthorHouse   09/04/2012

ISBN: 978-1-4772-2918-7 (sc)
ISBN: 978-1-4772-2919-4 (e)

Library of Congress Control Number: 2012914751

DEDICATION

I dedicate this book to my son Dan, whose support, insightful ideas and positive attitude gave me the inspiration to write this book, to my son Will, whose support, thoughtful perspective and timely assistance allowed me to complete this book, and to my husband, Mike, whose wisdom, constant encouragement and confidence in me kept me focused throughout this project. You have all been with me every step of the way, and I am filled with love and gratitude.

I also dedicate this book to all children with food allergies, I am in awe of the resolve and resilience with which you approach every challenge; to their families, I am constantly impressed, but never surprised, by your unwavering energy, perseverance and passion, and to the dedicated school personnel who partner with these families and strive to make school a safe environment where all students are able to participate fully in their academic and extra-curricular programs.

Food Allergies:
A Recipe For Success At School

**Information, Recommendations and Inspiration
for Families and School Personnel**

CONTENTS

ACKNOWLEDGEMENTS

I would like to thank the following individuals for generously sharing their expertise, comments and support, which I found invaluable in the writing of this book. Their interest in improving the quality of life of students with food allergies is respectfully acknowledged and greatly appreciated.

Michael C. Young, M.D., Assistant Clinical Professor of Pediatrics, Harvard Medical School; Allergist, Children's Hospital, Boston, Massachusetts, and at South Shore Allergy & Asthma Specialists, South Weymouth, Massachusetts; Author, *The Peanut Allergy Answer Book, Second Edition.*

Jennifer LeBovidge, Ph.D., Psychologist, Children's Hospital, Boston, Massachusetts.

Ray Wallace, Attorney, Disability and Education Rights, Wallace Law Office, P.C., Canton, Massachusetts.

Alan B. Dewey, Assistant Superintendent for Student Services, Canton Public Schools, Canton, Massachusetts.

Sharon Schumack, Director of Education Programs, Asthma & Allergy Foundation of America, New England Chapter, Needham, Massachusetts.

Judi McAuliffe, RN, NCSN, Nurse Leader, Pembroke Public Schools, Pembroke, Massachusetts.

Gail Kelley, RN, Nurse Leader, Dedham Public Schools, Dedham, Massachusetts

Terri McDonough, BSN, RN, Middle School Nurse, Hingham Public Schools, Hingham, Massachusetts.

Laurel Francoeur, Parent, Woburn, Massachusetts.

Fiona Murphy, Parent, Walpole, Massachusetts.

Rachel Butler, Parent, Hingham, Massachusetts, and former Editor-in-Chief, Asthma Magazine.

I am honored to have had your assistance and grateful to you all.

FOREWORD

With the continued increase in childhood food allergies in the U.S. over the past 25 years, schools are faced with a growing population of students at risk for severe, potentially life-threatening reactions. In the early 1990's, initial studies of near-fatal and fatal food anaphylaxis showed that for children, 80% of these reactions occurred in school settings. Subsequent studies examining the readiness of schools to prevent and manage students with food allergies identified significant deficiencies in all phases of management, from having no treatment plans, poor availability of emergency medications, to knowledge gaps on the part of parents, school staff and policy makers. Contributing to this difficult situation was the lack of scientific studies to inform guidelines and recommendations for the right thing to do for students with food allergies. Fortunately, by the early 2000's, studies did appear, proving the importance of early administration of epinephrine for treatment of anaphylaxis, examining effectiveness of cleaning methods in removal of allergen and showing low relative risks of anaphylaxis from skin contacts and inhalation exposures to peanut allergen—all relevant to the prevention, management and treatment plans of food allergic children in school settings. Subsequently, guidelines for the management of food allergies in schools have been developed and published. Despite these advances however, implementing these recommendations in real life is not easy, as many parents, school staff, nurses and physicians will attest!

Jan Hanson and her consulting group, Educating for Food Allergies, LLC (EFFA) was created more than 10 years ago to help families, schools, and the general public understand and overcome the problems facing the food allergic child in the school setting. Jan and EFFA have helped numerous families with individualized planning, assisted schools and communities with policy decisions, and educated school nurses, medical providers and the lay public with useful educational programs. Jan brings her wealth of knowledge and experience to writing this unique and pioneering book, the first book to specifically deal with all facets of food allergy management in schools. The book provides easy to understand summaries of the medical information, and an excellent review of the legal aspects of food allergies and schools nowhere else to be found. It is highlighted by real cases from Jan's practice. The practical information on formulating individual health care plans is invaluable. In writing this book, Jan Hanson has made an important contribution and every person involved in the care of school children with food allergies will benefit from reading it.

Michael C. Young, M.D.
Children's Hospital Boston, Division of Allergy & Immunology
Harvard Medical School
Author, *The Peanut Allergy Answer Book, Second Edition*

"We must remember that we cannot separate health from the ability to learn. The two must go together."

Surgeon General Antonia Novella, US Department of Health & Human Services, 1992

CHAPTER ONE

UNDERSTANDING FOOD ALLERGIES

Food allergy. These two words, said together, were rarely spoken in everyday conversation just twenty years ago. Not so today. It seems that everyone knows at least one person with a food allergy, whether that person is a neighbor, a friend's child, a student in your son or daughter's class, a niece or a nephew, or perhaps it is your own child. Food allergies are a growing phenomenon with no sign of abating. Food allergies have become, directly or indirectly, a part of the world in which we live. These two words, when spoken, rarely evoke a response of indifference. They do, however, often provoke many questions. Although there is much we still need to learn about food allergies, the information provided in this chapter will give an overview of what is known today about this complex health issue.

Current Statistics

Research studies looking at the epidemiology of food allergies became more prevalent during the 1990's, and they have continued worldwide since that time. The information revealed as a result of these studies allows us to develop a better understanding of what exactly food allergies are, and how we might be affected by them. A look at statistics over recent years demonstrates that the number of children with food allergies in the United States is growing at an alarming rate. A 2004 study in the *Journal of School Nursing* found that there was a 44% increase in the number of children at school with food allergies over the previous five years. In Massachusetts, an Essential School Health Services report demonstrated that from June 2007 to September 2008, there were a total of 16,365 students with a food allergy enrolled in 102 school districts. A recent study published in the July, 2011 issue of the medical journal, *Pediatrics*, reported that in the United States today, food allergies affect 6 million children under the age of 18. For school-aged children in the U.S., that means 8%, or one out of every thirteen children, will be diagnosed with some type of a food allergy. These statistics reflect a significantly higher number of children who have food allergies than were reported previously in similar studies.

Children are not only developing food allergies, they are also experiencing allergic reactions to food while at school. In a 2001 study by noted allergists and researchers Scott Sicherer, M.D. and Hugh Sampson, M.D., it was reported that 84% of students with a food allergy had an allergic reaction while in a school setting. Further evidence of this is found in the results of a 2005 study reported in *Pediatrics*, which demonstrated that 16-18% of children who had a food allergy experienced a food-allergic reaction during the school day. Data from the US Peanut and Tree Nut Allergy Registry indicate that 79% of allergic reactions to food occurred in the classroom, and 12% occurred in the cafeteria. Children are also having severe and life threatening reactions to their food allergens. In a Data Health Brief published by the Massachusetts Department of Public Health, it was revealed that from August, 2007 to July, 2008, 44% of anaphylactic reactions requiring epinephrine at school were caused by food. Tragically, children are also experiencing fatal reactions to their food allergens while at school. In a groundbreaking study by Dr. Hugh Sampson in 1992, it was determined that four out of six deaths from food-induced anaphylaxis occurred in the school setting. Another disturbing study in 2007 found that 50% of fatal food-allergic reactions among college-aged students occurred on the college campus. To view food allergies as a significant health concern would be appropriate.

Food Allergy Defined

We know that it can take only an infinitesimal amount of food to which we are allergic to cause an allergic reaction. It was reported in a 2008 study published in the *Journal of Allergy and Clinical Immunology* that over a two month period of time, 20,821 individuals visited a hospital emergency room due to a food-allergic reaction. This is an astounding number of people who experienced a traumatic, physical event. What exactly happens to someone when a food is eaten to which that person is allergic? The following information is intended to provide a basic understanding of the body's physiological response during a food-allergic reaction.

A True Food Allergy

Our body's immune system is designed to keep us healthy by protecting us from such things as harmful bacteria and viruses. For a person with a true food allergy, the immune system, in essence, misreads the information it receives. In other words, it mistakenly identifies the protein in the food to which the person is allergic as being harmful. For example, if someone is allergic to peanuts, the first time that individual ingests a peanut, the body red flags peanut protein as a foreign protein and in response, produces proteins called "IgE antibodies" that will recognize peanut protein if it enters the body again. These IgE antibodies attach themselves to mast cells, located in tissue found throughout the body, such as in the nose, throat, skin, lungs and gastrointestinal system, and to basophils, found in blood which circulates throughout the body, resulting in what is called "sensitization". These sensitized mast cells and basophils are now ready to recognize peanut protein when it enters the person's body again. If the person does eat peanut a second time, these sensitized mast cells and basophils spring into action by attaching to the food protein, in this case peanut protein. This action triggers the mast cells and basophils to release chemicals, such as histamine, which in turn causes the symptoms of an allergic reaction. The release of histamine happens very quickly, usually within five minutes of when the food protein (allergen) binds to the

IgE antibodies located on these mast cells and basophils, and can continue for thirty minutes to an hour. Whatever food a person is allergic to, whether it is peanuts, tree nuts, shellfish, milk, mustard, sesame seeds, mango, etc., the second time that food is ingested, the process of an allergic reaction as described above, will be put into motion.

A Food Intolerance

For people who have a food intolerance, as opposed to a true food allergy, the body's immune system is not involved and IgE antibodies are not produced. Rather, this is a metabolic disorder which does not allow the body to properly digest the food being consumed. Lactose intolerance is an example of a food intolerance. For someone who is lactose intolerant, the person is unable to break down lactose, which is a sugar present in milk products. If milk enters the body, the person would most likely experience an adverse physical reaction which can cause considerable discomfort, such as an upset stomach, abdominal bloating and other gastrointestinal symptoms.

Diagnosis of a Food Allergy

Consultation with a board-certified allergist is an important step to take when food seems to cause unwanted, adverse reactions, and our health, or that of a loved one, is being compromised. Your allergist will take a thorough medical history which will allow him or her to gather important information in order to make a diagnosis. During this appointment, you will be asked to describe: the symptoms being experienced, how long after eating the food do symptoms appear, if there are any specific foods which seem to trigger the reaction, and whether or not any family members have been diagnosed with an allergic disease, such as hayfever, eczema or asthma. Often, in conjunction with a medical history, diagnostic tests such as skin tests and blood tests will be performed to help diagnose a food allergy. In the skin prick test, a tiny amount of food extract is placed on the skin and then is gently "pricked" to allow it to reach below the top layer of the skin. The person will develop a red itchy hive on the area of the skin being tested if he is allergic to the food being tested. For blood tests, such as the ImmunoCAP test, blood is drawn and then examined in a laboratory to determine if IgE antibodies are being made to a specific food protein. Because it is possible to have a false positive result from either of these types of testing, your allergist may recommend that an oral food challenge test be performed in a medical setting in order to confirm whether or not the food, when eaten, causes an allergic reaction.

An excellent resource to further understand the diagnosis of a true food allergy is a publication issued by the *National Institute for Allergy and Infectious Disease (NIAID)*, entitled, **"Guidelines for the Diagnosis and Management of Food Allergy in the United States. Summary for Patients, Families, and Caregivers".**

Symptoms of an Allergic Reaction

When a person with a food allergy is exposed to one of his allergens, there are many different symptoms which may occur. The symptoms which develop during an allergic reaction will depend on which body system(s) has become involved, such as the skin, the gastrointestinal system (stomach and intestines), the respiratory system, and/or the cardiovascular system. A person having an allergic reaction will experience some of the symptoms listed below, but not necessarily all of them. It is also important to understand that the symptoms you have during one allergic reaction may be different than those you experience during a subsequent reaction. Similarly, while one reaction may be mild, your next reaction might be severe and life-threatening. Symptoms may start off very mild in nature but could progress to a severe reaction very rapidly, sometimes within minutes. Unfortunately, at this point in time, there is no way to predict which symptoms will develop after exposure to an offending allergen, or how severe or mild the reaction will be. Therefore, having the knowledge required to 1.) recognize symptoms of an allergic reaction, and 2.) understand that the symptoms being observed may progress rapidly to anaphylaxis, becomes critical, because it will promote better decision making in response to this type of an emergency, and help to insure that the appropriate medical intervention will be accessed quickly.

The Skin

When the skin is involved during an allergic reaction, symptoms might include itchy, red hives, and swelling (called edema) of the area of the skin that has come in contact with the allergen—most commonly in the lips, tongue and/or eyelids. If the person has a pre-existing condition of eczema, then he might experience an eczema flare during the allergic reaction. If you eat a food to which you are allergic, some of the first symptoms you may notice might be an itchy mouth and lips, and redness and swelling in that area. Although most allergic reactions begin with skin symptoms, this is not always the case. It is interesting to note that during some food-induced allergic reactions, skin symptoms do not develop at all.

The Gastrointestinal System

The gastrointestinal system refers to the stomach and intestines. When a food allergen has reached these areas of the body, a person may experience abdominal cramps, gas, nausea, vomiting and diarrhea.

The Respiratory System

During an allergic reaction, the respiratory system may produce symptoms such as a stuffy or runny nose, and sneezing or coughing, often repetitively. In addition, a person may have difficulty swallowing. Children may describe this sensation as feeling like there is something caught in their throat. It is also possible to hear a change in the way the person's voice normally sounds, such as being either higher or lower or perhaps "squeaky". Symptoms of asthma, such as wheezing or shortness of breath, may develop. The onset of respiratory symptoms often signals that the allergic reaction is becoming more severe.

The Cardiovascular System

When the cardiovascular system is involved, the reaction has become severe and is life threatening. Symptoms may include paleness, a bluish tint of the skin, dizziness, feeling faint, confusion, a weak pulse and a drop in blood pressure. It is also possible for a person to lose consciousness when blood circulation is affected. People who have experienced these types of symptoms have described feeling a sense of impending doom.

SYMPTOMS OF AN ALLERGIC REACTION

Skin
Hives
Swelling of the Affected Area (often the lips, tongue, eyelids)
Itchy, Red Rash (Eczema Flare)

Gastrointestinal

Cramps	Diarrhea
Nausea	Vomiting

Respiratory

Itchy, watery eyes	Difficulty Swallowing
Coughing	Tightness in the Chest
Runny or Stuffy Nose	Shortness of Breath
Sneezing (often repetitive)	Wheezing
Change in Voice	

Cardiovascular

Dizziness	Skin turns Pale or Bluish
Confusion	Chest Pain
Feeling Faint, Weak	Drop in Blood Pressure

Anaphylaxis

The most severe form of an allergic reaction is called "anaphylaxis". A reaction of this nature can be life threatening and cause death. The symptoms of an anaphylactic reaction usually appear within five to thirty minutes after someone has been exposed to the allergen. It is possible for symptoms of an anaphylactic reaction to subside after treatment, only to reappear with a vengeance four to eight hours later. This is referred to as a biphasic reaction and statistically, 5-20% of all cases of anaphylaxis are biphasic. For a very long time there was no consensus on exactly how anaphylaxis should be defined. As a result, there is speculation that incidences of anaphylaxis have been under-recognized and under-reported. In July, 2005, the National Institute of Allergy and Infectious Disease (NIAID) and the Food Allergy & Anaphylaxis Network (FAAN) convened for a second time in order to define anaphylaxis in a way that would be agreed upon across organizations and specialties of medicine. As a result of the concerted efforts of these two organizations, a definition was finally agreed upon at this second symposium. The definition that is to be used by both medical professionals and the non-medical community is:

"Anaphylaxis is a serious allergic reaction that is rapid in onset and may cause death."

This group also agreed upon specific ***DIAGNOSTIC CRITERIA*** to be used. They are:

ANAPHYLAXIS IS HIGHLY LIKELY TO OCCUR WHEN ANY ONE OF THE FOLLOWING OCCURS (WITHIN MINUTES TO HOURS):

1. An individual has acute onset of symptoms (minutes to several hours) involving the skin (generalized hives, pruritis

or flushing) and/or swelling of the lips, tongue or uvula, *and* at least one of the following:

a. Respiratory difficulty (eg. Dyspnea, wheeze-bronchospasm, stridor, reduced PEF, hypoxemia)

b. Reduced BP or associated symptoms of end-organ dysfunction (eg. Hypotonia (collapse), syncope, incontinence)

2. An individual was exposed to a ***suspected allergen*** and two or more of the following occur within minutes to several hours:

a. Involvement of the skin-mucosal tissue (eg. Generalized hives, itch-flush, swollen lips-tongue-uvula)

b. Respiratory difficulty (eg. Dyspnea, wheeze-bronchospasm, stridor, reduced PEF, hypoxemia)

c. Reduced BP or associated symptoms (eg. Hypotonia (collapse), syncope, incontinence)

d. Persistent gastrointestinal symptoms (eg. cramping, abdominal pain, vomiting)

3. An individual has had a ***known exposure*** to an allergen and experiences a reduced blood pressure within minutes to several hours:

a. Infants and children: low systolic Blood Pressure (age specific) or greater than 30% decrease in systolic Blood Pressure

b. Adults: systolic Blood Pressure of less than 90mmHg or greater than 30% decrease from that person's baseline

Epinephrine should be given immediately when the above criteria are met **_or_** for an individual with a history of life-threatening reactions who has had exposure to an allergen and begins to have symptoms quickly, even if they are mild.

(Source: 2nd National Institute of Allergy and Infectious Disease/FAAN Anaphylaxis Symposium July, 2005)

Please refer to the Supplemental Materials for a printable version of the NIAID Anaphylaxis Diagnostic Criteria.

An anaphylactic reaction should be regarded as a serious medical event. Current data indicates that the incidence of anaphylaxis in the United Sates is occurring in numbers that justify great concern. In an editorial printed in a recent *Journal of Allergy and Clinical Immunology*, titled, "Anaphylaxis epidemic: Fact or fiction?" the authors concluded that the rate of anaphylaxis in the U.S. has increased so much in recent years, that the term "epidemic" may be appropriately applied. Support for this conclusion is found in the 2008 study referenced earlier in this chapter which looked at the incidence of food-allergic reactions seen at a hospital ER over a period of two months. This study also found that there were 2,333 ER visits for anaphylaxis over that same two month period of time. In yet another study, it was determined that food allergies, primarily peanut and tree nut allergies, account for 150-200 deaths annually. School-aged children are not immune to these morbid statistics, as was evidenced by the 2012 death of a first grade student in a Virginia school due to food-induced anaphylaxis. Current data indicates that teenagers and young adults experience the greatest number of fatalities due to anaphylaxis caused by food allergy.

Risk Factors for Anaphylaxis

There are certain factors which increase the risk of anaphylaxis for an individual who has a food allergy. Current data indicates that people who have either a *peanut or tree nut allergy* are at a higher risk for having anaphylaxis. A *previous history* of having had anaphylaxis is another risk factor, and an individual with *asthma* is also at higher risk for anaphylaxis. It appears that the *teenage years* are also a significant factor linked to an increased risk of anaphylaxis. A *delay* in receiving prompt treatment with epinephrine also increases the risk for anaphylaxis and fatality.

Risk Factors for Anaphylaxis

► A previous history of anaphylaxis   ► Asthma

► Peanut or Tree Nut Allergy

► Delay in Treating with Epinephrine

► The Teenage Years

Treatment

Epinephrine is the treatment of choice for anaphylaxis, and it is most effective when given as soon as the symptoms of anaphylaxis have been recognized. Everyone who is diagnosed with a life threatening food allergy should carry epinephrine with them at all times. There are currently four epinephrine auto-injector devices available on the market. The DEY Company makes an epinephrine auto-injector device sold under the name EpiPen® and EpiPen® Jr. to deliver this life-saving medicine. They are packaged as a single dose or with two auto-injectors in one box. Two additional options for epinephrine auto-injectors are made by Shionogi Pharma, Inc. and are sold under the names Twinject® and Adrenaclick® (Twinject® was previously manufactured by Verus Pharmaceuticals, Inc.). The Twinject® device contains two delivery mechanisms for epinephrine; the first dose is delivered as an auto-injector device, however the second dose, if needed, must be administered manually as an injection. Adrenaclick® is sold in either a single dose or as a twin pack. As of May, 2010, Shionogi Pharma contracted with Greenstone Pharmaceuticals to manufacture a generic epinephrine auto-injector, which may be substituted for the Adrenaclick®. Currently, there is no generic epinephrine auto-injector device which may be substituted for the EpiPen® or EpiPen® Jr. Please be aware that each brand of epinephrine auto-injector device will have different instructions for its use. The EpiPen® and EpiPen® Jr. are the devices most commonly prescribed, and therefore, we will focus on their use for the remainder of this chapter.

The epinephrine auto-injector made by the DEY Company is available by prescription in two doses, which are based on body weight: .15mg of epinephrine, typically prescribed for children 33-66 pounds (the EpiPen® Jr.), and .3mg of epinephrine, typically prescribed for individuals 66 pounds and more (the EpiPen®). The allergist will determine the appropriate dose based on the patient's weight and medical history. The EpiPen® device is easy to administer and was designed to be used by people who do not have any medical training. Instructions for the proper technique in using this medication delivery system should be discussed with your doctor. Written instructions may also be found inside the packaging. The EpiPen® should be administered in the muscle of the outer thigh because that is where the medicine will be absorbed most quickly. Although not optimal, it is designed to go through clothes if there is concern that not enough time exists to remove clothing. When using the EpiPen®, it is important not to put your thumb over the end of the device, because that will interfere with the delivery of the medicine. When the auto-injector has been activated, remember to count to ten SLOWLY before you remove it away from the person's thigh. This will help to insure that all of the medicine has been delivered. The correct dose of the medicine has been administered if the needle tip is extended and the window area of the EpiPen® is obscured.

It is important to understand that epinephrine will not cause any serious side effects in an otherwise healthy, young person. After receiving epinephrine, however, an individual may develop a rapid heart beat, an elevated blood pressure, a headache, nausea and feel "shaky" as if he or she had too much coffee. Because the side effects of epinephrine are short-lived, they should resolve quickly. Once someone has been treated with epinephrine, it is very important to call 911 immediately, and inform them that the individual is experiencing "anaphylaxis". Using this word specifically will help the EMTs to recognize the seriousness of the emergency, and respond appropriately. Although most states have ambulances equipped with epinephrine and emergency first responders trained to administer it, it is a good idea to check and make sure this is the case in your community. When an individual has been treated for anaphylaxis in an emergency room, it is important that the person remain in the hospital setting for a full four hours, just in case symptoms return due to a biphasic reaction. If treated and released before four hours have passed, it is strongly recommended that the individual remain in the waiting room for the full four hours.

The effects of epinephrine last anywhere from ten to twenty minutes. Having **two** epinephrine auto-injectors on hand *at all times* is a good idea for two reasons: 1.) as a back-up should anything go wrong during the delivery of the medicine, and 2.) to use to deliver a second dose of epinephrine if the first dose is ineffective, or if the person were to experience a biphasic reaction. The American Academy of Pediatrics advises that a second dose of epinephrine may be given as soon as five minutes after the first dose was administered if it was not effective in reversing symptoms, or if symptoms continue to worsen. If all you have is an expired EpiPen®, USE IT! The medicine may not be full-strength, but it is definitely better than nothing. Epinephrine needs to be stored in a temperature-controlled environment, and should not be exposed to temperatures higher than 86 degrees or lower than 59 degrees. Storing the EpiPen® or EpiPen® Jr in an insulated bag is recommended, because it will help to maintain an acceptable temperature for the medicine. Thankfully, insulated lunch bags, which are relatively inexpensive, come in a variety of sizes and colors, and are usually sold in pharmacies and a variety of retail stores.

Questions arise periodically regarding whether there is a role for antihistamines in treating an allergic reaction and anaphylaxis. Antihistamines will NOT stop the symptoms of anaphylaxis. An antihistamine may, however, be used as a *secondary* treatment after epinephrine has been administered. Used in this manner, antihistamines will help relieve skin symptoms such as hives and itchiness. Seek the advice of your allergist before an allergic reaction or anaphylaxis occurs, to determine how best to treat it.

The Joint Task Force on Practice Parameters, a group comprised of the American Academy of Allergy, Asthma & Immunology (AAAAI), the American College of Allergy, Asthma & Immunology (ACAAI), and the Joint Council of Allergy, Asthma & Immunology, developed practice parameters to assist physicians in the diagnosis and management of anaphylaxis. The parameters are titled, "The Diagnosis and Management of Anaphylaxis Practice Parameter: 2010 Update". Refer to the AAAAI website for more information: www.aaaai.org.

Another important resource produced in 2010 that offers guidance to healthcare professionals in the management of their patients with food allergy is written by The National Institute of Allergy and Infectious Diseases (NIAID), and is titled: "Guidelines for the Diagnosis and Management of Food Allergy in the United States: Report of the NIAID-Sponsored Expert Panel". A summary of these guidelines is available for patients, families and caregivers, and can be found on their website: www.niaid.nih.gov.

Foods That Cause Allergic Reactions

What foods are responsible for causing allergic reactions? First, it is important to understand that *any* food is capable of causing an allergic reaction and anaphylaxis. There are eight foods, however, know as **"the Big Eight"** which are primarily responsible for causing the majority of allergic reactions to food in the U.S. They are: peanuts, tree nuts, milk, eggs, wheat, soy, fish and shellfish. Peanuts, tree nuts, egg and milk are the most common food allergens which cause problems for children. Seed allergies are becoming much more prevalent, and more and more children are being diagnosed with sesame, poppy, sunflower, mustard and cottonseed allergies.

THE BIG EIGHT

Peanuts*	Milk*
Tree Nuts*	Eggs*
Wheat	Fish
Soy	Shellfish

* Most common for children

Peanut and Tree Nut Allergy

Peanuts: Recent studies indicate that 1-2% of children in the US are allergic to peanuts and tree nuts. Peanuts are actually a member of the legume family of vegetables, and are not actually nuts. Peanuts, also sometimes referred to as "goobers", "groundnuts", and "earthnuts", have a very high protein content. In addition to whole peanuts, peanut butter, peanut flour, and peanut oil (arachis oil), peanuts can be found in candies containing peanuts, in some chilis, brown gravies and barbecue sauces, egg rolls, enchilada sauce, Chinese foods, Satay sauces, vegetarian foods, meat products, granola bars, mandelonas (peanuts soaked in almond flavoring), many pastries, cookies and baked goods.

<u>Tree Nuts</u>: Tree nuts include: almonds, cashews, filberts and hazelnuts, macadamia nuts, chestnuts, mandelonas, pecans, pistachios, walnuts (Black and English), butternuts (a white walnut), pralines, pinenuts (pinynon), brazil nuts and hickory nuts. In addition to nut flours, nut butters and nut oils, tree nuts can be found in candies, nougat, marzipan (almond paste), pesto, many baked and dessert items, cereals, granolas, sauces, salads and salad dressings. Tree nuts may also be used to flavor liqueurs, such as Amaretto (almond) and Frangelico (hazelnut). Although coconut may be defined as a nut, a true coconut allergy is relatively uncommon. Despite their names, it is interesting to note that water chestnuts and nutmeg are not nuts, and therefore, need not be restricted for tree-nut allergic individuals.

Both peanuts and tree nuts are often used as ingredients in birdseeds, bean bags, shampoos, soaps, skin creams, bath oils and cosmetics. Gourmet peanut and nut oils are typically cold-pressed, and as a result, the protein in these products is capable of causing an allergic reaction in people who have these allergies. On the other hand, most peanut and nut oils produced in the United States are heat-processed, and therefore, the protein in the oils become denatured making them incapable of causing an allergic reaction. The decision whether to ingest these heat-processed oils should occur however, only after discussion with your allergist.

Peanut allergy receives a great deal of attention and research. This may be due in large part because peanut allergy is persistent and in most cases, will not be outgrown. It is often responsible for severe allergic reactions and it can significantly affect the individual and his/her family's quality of life. An important study which investigated the prevalence of peanut and tree nut allergy in the United States, first in 1997, and then again in 2002, found that the rate of peanut allergy in children had doubled over that time period. Information gathered in 2008 as an eleven year follow-up to this study indicated that self-reported peanut and tree nut allergies in children has increased significantly since 1997, and has, in fact, tripled. This information becomes particularly significant when it is coupled with the fact that peanuts and tree nuts are the foods responsible for 90% of fatal reactions. To make matters worse, ingesting only a minute amount of food may cause an allergic reaction. For people with peanut allergy, for example, it takes as little as 2 mg, which equals 1/250 of a peanut, to provoke symptoms of an allergic reaction. It is difficult to imagine that such an infinitesimal piece of food can be capable of wreaking such havoc with the human body.

Investigation into the epidemiology of peanut allergy has revealed some important information. First, it appears that how a peanut is cooked or processed influences its allergenicity. Research indicates that the process of dry roasting peanuts increases their allergenic properties. This fact is significant when we understand that in the United States peanut butter is made by using dry, roasted peanuts. Conversely, in China, despite the consumption of large quantities of peanuts, there is no evidence of widespread peanut allergy. This may be explained by the fact that in China, most peanuts that are eaten are boiled, rather than roasted. Genetics also plays a significant role in the development of peanut allergy. There is scientific evidence to support that a family history of allergic diseases influences a child's risk of developing allergic diseases, such as food allergy. Furthermore, children have a 7% risk of developing a peanut allergy if they have a sibling who has a peanut allergy. In addition, if a child has eczema, especially in the first six months of life, there is a stronger likelihood of developing a food allergy to peanut, egg and milk.

Milk Allergy

Cow's milk is the most common food allergy for young children. It is estimated that 2.5% of youngsters under the age of three have an allergy to milk. In addition to the cow's milk that people drink, milk protein is also found in other related foods, such as cheeses and cottage cheese, butter, margarine, yogurt, sour cream, whipped cream, sweetened condensed milk, evaporated milk, powdered milk and ice cream. Milk products are used in coffee whiteners, custards, puddings, pastries, some luncheon meats, hot dogs, sausages, pasta dishes, pancakes, waffles and French toast. It appears that some individuals with a milk allergy can tolerate milk if it has been sufficiently heated or cooked, such as milk found in cooked or baked goods, for example. It has been reported that approximately 70% of children with a milk allergy are able to eat baked goods safely when the milk has been extensively heated. Families of a child with a milk allergy should not attempt this, however, without prior discussion and approval from their allergist.

Egg Allergy

Egg allergy is common and is found in approximately 1-2% of children. There has been documentation of a link between the development of eczema and the development of egg allergy in infants and children. In addition to its whole form, egg, which can have either a white or brown shell, can be found as an ingredient in a multitude of products, such as breads, cakes and other baked goods, bagels, souffles, waffles, pancakes, French toast, macaroni, mayonnaise, meringue, marshmallows, custards, pretzels and some ice creams, sauces, dressings and pasta dishes. There are some individuals with an egg allergy who can not safely eat a raw egg, but are able to ingest cooked eggs without developing symptoms of an allergic reaction. Again, this should not be attempted without the allergist's approval.

Wheat Allergy

In the U.S., one child in every 250 children will develop a wheat allergy. Wheat, which contains a high amount of gluten, can be found in such foods as breads, pastas, cereals, flour, baked goods, wheat germ oil, pilafs, semolina, ice cream cones and pizza dough. Wheat can also be found in modeling dough, which is sometimes used in school projects. It is interesting to note that celiac disease, which causes the body's immune system to respond abnormally to gluten, does not involve the production of IgE antibodies. Therefore, celiac disease is not typically defined as a true food allergy.

Soy Allergy

Soy is another common food allergen and affects 0.4% of children in the U.S. Infant formulas that contain soy protein are often recommended for infants who are allergic to milk. Soybean, also known as "edamame", is a member of the legume family. Soybean oil is frequently used as a vegetable oil for cooking and baking. Soy products may be found in soy sauce, margarines and shortenings, tofu, canned tuna, cereals, crackers, in many processed meats, and is often used in salads, salad dressings, sauces and soups.

Fish and Shellfish Allergy

Fish and shellfish allergies, which can cause severe allergic reactions, are more common for adults than for children. It is estimated that 6.6 million Americans have a fish or shellfish allergy.

Fish: Approximately 50% of individuals who have a fish allergy will have allergies to more than one fish. The word "fish" refers to fish with fins, regardless of whether their habitat is freshwater or saltwater. There are many varieties of fish, including catfish, trout, perch, haddock, cod, red snapper, tilapia, hake, halibut, salmon, flounder and tuna. Fish, fish oils and fish stock can be found in sauces, Worcestershire sauce, chowders, soups, pasta and salad dishes and some dressings.

Shellfish: Shellfish may be divided into three categories:
1.) Crustaceans, which include crab, crayfish, lobster and shrimp, 2.) Mollusks, which include abalone, scallops, clams, mussels, and oysters, and 3.) Cephalopods, which include octopus and squid (calamari). Shellfish can be found in foods and prepared dishes

similar to those listed under fish, and may also be found in some brands of imitation shellfish.

Routes of Allergen Exposure

There are many ways in which a person may be exposed to one of their food allergens. It is important to understand how a child might come in contact with their allergen(s), and the risks associated with each route of exposure.

INGESTION

As one might expect, eating a food to which we are allergic will undoubtedly trigger symptoms of an allergic reaction. We also know that it can take relatively small amounts of a food protein to which we are allergic to cause a reaction. The task of successfully avoiding food allergens requires constant effort and relentless ingredient label reading. With the passing of the Food Allergen Labeling and Consumer Protection Act (FALCPA) into law in 2006, thanks to the hard work of the Food Allergy & Anaphylaxis Network and the Food Allergy Initiative, avoiding food allergens has become a little bit easier. If a food sold within the U.S. contains a "major food allergen", which is defined as one of "the Big Eight", namely milk, egg, wheat, soy, peanuts, tree nuts, fish and shellfish, it must appear on the product's label in clear language. Foods that are not included in "the Big Eight", however, do not have to be specifically declared. For example, although sesame and garlic might be foods used in the "natural flavorings" of an ingredient list, they might not be clearly identified as such. In addition, FALCPA does not regulate allergen advisory labels on packages, but rather instructs manufacturers to be truthful in what is printed. A recent study investigating possible ambiguities with advisory labeling found that a total of 25 different types of advisory language exist, a fact which presents a definite challenge for the consumer. This study also points out that currently there is not a FALCPA requirement to alert consumers when a new ingredient has been added to a food product.

Another study was conducted to look at advisory labels which indicate the possibility of the presence of peanuts in a packaged food. Labels investigated included such language as "may contain peanuts" and "made in a shared facility with peanuts". It was determined that out of 400 samples tested with these types of advisory labeling, 10% actually did contain peanut protein. This study also found that peanut protein may be present regardless of which type of advisory language is used. Because of this, it is strongly recommended that individuals with a peanut allergy do not consume any food products that contain allergen advisory labels which indicate that peanuts might be present. Although much improvement has been made regarding language used for food ingredient lists found on products manufactured in the U.S., additional progress is needed in this area in order to allow individuals with food allergies to be able to make better-informed, and thus safer choices, when purchasing food items.

Despite concerted efforts, accidental ingestion of a food allergen can happen. Results from a 2009 research study found that over a twelve month period of time, milk-allergic children in this study had a significant number of accidental ingestions to milk, some so severe that hospitalization was required.

Example of exposure to a food allergen through ingestion at school: At an after-school care program, a project making gingerbread houses was planned by the teacher. The teacher, aware that there was a Kindergarten student in the class allergic to eggs, did not use any whole eggs for the project, and based on that, believed that the project was safe for her egg-allergic student. Unfortunately, Marshmallow Fluff®, which contains eggs as an ingredient, was one of the foods used to create "snow" on the houses. The student, upon finding marshmallow stuck to his hands, requested permission to go to the bathroom to wash it off. He was told that he could "clean" his hands by licking off the marshmallow. The project took place at the very end of the day. When the boy's mother arrived to pick him up, she found his face swollen and covered in hives, symptoms of an allergic reaction that had apparently gone unnoticed by the teacher. Upon learning what had transpired, she raced him to the hospital Emergency Room, where he was treated with epinephrine and was eventually released. _Lesson Learned_: Never assume that a food is safe! Foods should not be eaten unless an ingredient list can, and has been, carefully read to determine that no allergens exist. This same procedure should be followed whenever foods will be used in classroom projects. Good, clear communication between the teacher and parent can help to eliminate accidents from happening. It is also critical that epinephrine be administered after ingestion of a known allergen, and that 911 is called immediately.

**You Should Know**: A 2006 study investigated ways in which to reduce peanut protein in the saliva after peanut butter has been consumed. They concluded with 95% confidence that 90% of people who eat peanut butter will have no detectable peanut in their mouths if they subsequently 1.) eat a peanut-free meal and 2.) allow several hours to pass. They found this combination was actually more effective in reducing peanut protein in saliva than brushing teeth or chewing gum.

SKIN CONTACT

An allergic reaction may occur when an individual's allergen comes into contact with his/her skin. An exposure of this type may produce only skin symptoms, such as hives, redness and localized swelling. Allergic reactions of this nature are typically not serious, and may successfully be treated by giving the individual an antihistamine, in conjunction with washing the affected area with soap and water. Unfortunately, however, if the person's hands have touched the offending allergen and before being cleaned, the contaminated hands touch the eyes, nose and/or mouth, the allergen has now entered the individual's system through the mucous membranes. This scenario could initiate a systemic, and more serious allergic reaction.

In an effort to determine the risk of anaphylaxis caused by skin contact with peanut butter, researchers placed a small amount of peanut butter on the lower backs of the children enrolled in their study. The only symptoms seen, after an hour of observation, were hives on the lower back of only 1/3 of the subjects. In fact, the reactions were so mild, that no medicine of any kind was needed to treat the reactions. The results of the study indicated no significant risk of anaphylaxis from skin contact with peanut butter. The researchers noted, however, that larger amounts of peanut butter, for example, amounts that might be used during a classroom project (such as making bird feeders), could be an important variable in causing a significant allergic reaction.

Another research study which sought to find factors that influence the development of peanut allergy found that infants who have skin exposure to peanut oil are at an increased risk for developing peanut allergy. This study also identified eczema as another risk factor for developing peanut allergy, and theorized that peanut protein may enter the body through inflamed skin resulting from this condition. In a more recent study published in a 2009 *Journal of Allergy & Clinical Immunology*, it was determined that high levels of exposure to peanut in the environment for infants with eczema, especially during the first year of their lives, was a possible factor in increasing the risk of developing peanut allergy. The researchers suggest that when a household member eats a food containing peanuts, and then subsequently touches a surface, such as a table or chair within the house, the infant may later touch that same surface and become exposed to the peanut protein. The authors noted that peanut butter may pose a greater risk than other forms of peanut because it contains a high concentration of peanut protein and it is "sticky", which makes it easily transferred from a table surface to the skin.

Example of exposure of a food allergen through skin contact at school: A peanut-allergic student in elementary school developed symptoms of an allergic reaction, (hives and redness around the mouth, and swelling around the eyes) regularly after he used a computer during the lesson at school. He would be treated with an antihistamine by the school nurse, who would also wash the affected area. Although these did not develop into serious allergic reactions because they were recognized quickly and treated promptly, the effect of the antihistamine left the student drowsy and unable to concentrate. These side effects negatively impacted the student's ability to do his best work at school. *Lesson Learned*: It was determined that peanut butter residue, although not visible to the student or teacher, was probably being transferred from another non-allergic student who typically ate a peanut butter sandwich at lunch and then was assigned to use this same computer keyboard. The student with the peanut allergy had computer class later in the afternoon after this student. To avoid further allergic reactions due to skin exposure, the peanut-allergic student was assigned to the same computer for each lesson. Prior to his arrival, the teacher would wipe down the keyboard with a commercial wet wipe, and as a further precaution, the student would wash his hands after the lesson was completed. Once these procedures were implemented, he never experienced another allergic reaction associated with using the computer.

You Should Know: There are easy and effective ways to remove peanut residue so that exposure through skin contact may be greatly reduced. A 2004 study looked at effective ways in which to remove peanut residue from the hands and from table surfaces. Based on study results, washing with good old-fashioned bar or liquid soap and water is the most effective means of removing peanut residue from the hands. Commercial wet wipes were found to be a close second in productively removing peanut protein from the skin. However, alcohol-based, antibacterial hand sanitizers, such as Purell®, were found to leave detectable amounts of peanut, and should, therefore, not be considered as an effective method of peanut protein removal. This same study found that most household cleaning products should be effective in removing peanut residue from table surfaces; commercial products investigated that were particularly effective were: Formula 409®, Lysol Sanitizing Wipes® and Target® brand cleaner with bleach.

INHALATION

It is possible for tiny particles of a food to be released into the air and become airborne. This process may occur in several different ways. For example, boiling or steaming foods, such as milk or fish, will release the protein of that food into the air. Another way for a food protein to become airborne is when tiny particles of these foods are released into the air while the food is being eaten. This process can happen when foods such as peanuts or nuts are eaten. If someone were to inhale tiny protein particles of an allergenic food, he or she could experience an allergic reaction through what is called "inhalation exposure". Allergic symptoms resulting from inhalation are typically itchy eyes, runny nose, sneezing or coughing, and are similar to allergic symptoms from other airborne allergens, such as dust, pollen or animal dander. The school environment does present several scenarios where allergen exposure through inhalation may occur. Caution should be exercised in the planning of any projects which involve cooking or steaming of foods. Similar scrutiny should be applied to science experiments where food products are cooked or heated in an effort to analyze their various properties, for example. If a student will be present who is allergic to the food being investigated, then alternative foods should be selected which are safe for all students who will participate in the project.

Example of exposure to a food allergen through inhalation at school: A middle school student, who was highly allergic to peanuts and tree nuts, was assigned to a schedule of classrooms which would be maintained as peanut and nut free. One day as he sat at his desk, a bowl which had been used in a classroom not designated as nut-free, was being washed with hot water in the sink located in his room. As the bowl was washed, the student, who was seated within close proximity to the sink, began to develop hives on his face and swelling around his eyes. He went to the health office and was treated with an antihistamine by the nurse, where he remained under observation until his symptoms eventually resolved. It was later discovered that the bowl had contained an assortment of ingredients, including nuts and peanuts. ***Lesson Learned***: If it is determined that a specific food(s) should be restricted from a classroom due to a severe allergy, then all efforts should be made to insure that the food stays out of that classroom, for any reason.

You Should Know: A study conducted by Simonte, et al. examined reactions to the smell of peanut butter. Results of this study found that NO allergic symptoms result from the smell of peanut butter. The chemicals which cause the odor of peanuts are called Pyrazines. Because pyrazines do not contain any protein, which is necessary to cause an allergic reaction, the actual "smell" or odor of peanut butter can not cause a true allergic reaction. Inhaling airborne peanut protein particles from peanut flour or from pieces of a peanut, would, on the other hand, be capable of causing an allergic reaction due to inhalation exposure.

CROSS-CONTAMINATION

When one food comes into contact with another food, the proteins of each food will inevitably mix. When this happens, each food will then contain small amounts of the other food, although the presence of both foods may be invisible to the observer. The occurrence of this process is referred to as "cross-contamination". In a school setting, this is most likely to happen in the cafeteria, in a home economics or consumer science class, or in the classroom where allergenic snacks and/or lunch will be eaten. For example, if a food is being prepared on a counter, and prior to cleaning, another food is prepared on the same area of the counter, cross-contamination of the foods will likely occur. If a knife is used to cut one type of sandwich, and is then used to cut another type of sandwich, then again, cross-contamination of the foods will occur. In the classroom, if a child eats cheese and crackers at a table, and subsequently, another child, who happens to be allergic to milk, sits in the same location to eat his snack of grapes, it is possible for residue from the cheese and crackers to come into contact with the grapes. While the second child eats his safe snack of grapes, he may unknowingly ingest some cheese, and experience an allergic reaction due to cross-contamination of the foods present.

__Example of exposure to a food allergen through cross-contamination at school__: A thirteen year old student allergic to peanuts, dairy products and soybeans, and who also had asthma, wanted to have the opportunity to eat in her school cafeteria. She carefully checked with cafeteria staff to make sure that the French fries she hoped to eat, were safe for her. After being assured that they were safe, she purchased the French fries and proceeded to eat them. She very quickly began to experience the symptoms of an allergic reaction, but because she thought the food she was eating was safe, she believed the cause of her symptoms was her asthma. As her symptoms worsened, it became clear that epinephrine was needed. Unfortunately, there was a significant delay in receiving this medicine, first because she had misinterpreted her symptoms, but also because her EpiPen® was kept in her locker, which was a distance from the cafeteria. Tragically, this young student named Sabrina, died from anaphylaxis. It was determined that the tongs used to serve her the French fries had also been in contact with cheese present in the cafeteria kitchen. *Lesson Learned*: This horrific incident, which took place in Ontario, Canada, became the catalyst for the passing of Sabrina's Law, which took effect in Ontario in January, 2006. This law requires schools in Ontario to have policies in place for their students with life-threatening allergies, including preventing exposure to their allergens, and training implemented for school staff on how to manage life-threatening allergies.

You Should Know: Caution should be exercised regarding advisory labeling on food products, such as "May Contain . . .", "Made on Shared Equipment with . . .", "Made in a Shared Facility with . . ." etc., because the food may actually contain trace amounts of the allergen listed. A 2007 study presented by Hefle, et al. in the *Journal of Allergy and Clinical Immunology* which looked at the presence of peanuts and nuts found in products with advisory labeling, found that 10% of these products did, in fact, contain traces of peanuts and nuts. It is extremely important to read ingredient labels each and every time a food is purchased; ingredient lists change regularly and therefore constant vigilance is required.

MORE ABOUT FOOD ALLERGIES

The growing numbers of people being diagnosed with a food allergy, and in many cases multiple food allergies, has caused many important questions to be asked. Scientific research, which is ongoing, will help to provide much needed information to allow both the medical community and everyone affected by food allergy to develop a better understanding of this complex health issue. This increased knowledge will enable better decision making regarding the ways in which food allergies should be approached for optimal results, in terms of both its management and treatment.

►Why Are Food Allergies Increasing?

There are several different theories based on current research which offer possible explanations for why food allergies are on the rise. To date, however, no theories have been scientifically proven and universally accepted. The following are two theories of interest.

Theory One: The increase in food allergies may be due to environmental variables and is explained in what is called the **"Hygiene Hypothesis"**. The concept of this approach focuses on the idea that our society has evolved into being essentially "too clean". The twentieth century has produced many advances in science which have increased our chances of staying healthy. For example, we have witnessed the introduction of antibiotics, such as penicillin, which have allowed people to win what otherwise might have been a losing battle against serious bacterial infections. We have seen the benefit of immunizations to guard against illnesses caused by viruses and bacteria, such as those for tetanus, diphtheria, polio, for example. More recently, our fight against illness has expanded to include antibacterial soaps and hand sanitizers. Our homes have become more airtight in order to keep out cold and wet weather. It would certainly be fair to say that all of these advances have allowed most people to live healthier and longer lives. Unfortunately, the possible downside of this type of progress is the fact that the immune system, which is genetically programmed to detect and fight invading organisms intent on causing harm, such as germs, viruses, and bacteria, is left to find new targets, such as benign environmental and dietary allergens. For individuals with food allergy, the immune system mistakenly perceives the protein in the food as being harmful and consequently fights the food protein, which produces the symptoms of an allergic reaction.

Theory Two: The increase in peanut allergy, specifically, may be attributed to an infant's **exposure to peanut and peanut products through skin contact and inhalation**. Recent research conducted in 2008 hypothesizes that the development of peanut allergy may be a result of a combination of two, concurrent factors: 1.) avoidance of ingesting any peanut products during infancy and early childhood, and 2.) skin contact during infancy with peanut proteins found in the household environment, especially when it is found in large amounts. This appears to be particularly true for infants who suffer from eczema flares. Scientists involved in this study theorize that individuals who are subject to these two factors may have a reduced likelihood of developing the ability to eat peanuts safely. More research is required in order to support and further substantiate this premise.

Several other theories are currently under investigation in an attempt to determine if there are other variables which may play a role in the increasing incidence of food allergies. One possible variable that has gained attention is the role fats play in our diet. Research indicates that a reduced consumption of animal fats, combined with an increase of margarine and vegetable oils in our diets, has led to an increase in asthma, eczema and allergic rhinitis (hayfever). Another variable being investigated is whether too much or too little exposure to Vitamin D will influence the onset of allergic diseases. More research is needed in order to identify the efficacy of such variables in the development of food allergies.

▶Noteworthy Changes Made to Dietary Recommendations:

American Academy of Pediatrics (AAP) Committee on Nutrition (section on Allergy and Immunology): In 2000, the American Academy of Pediatrics published a Clinical Report regarding recommendations for nutritional guidelines meant to delay or prevent the development of atopic diseases in children. In 2008, the AAP rescinded these recommendations due to a lack of evidence to support them. The 2008 report did, however, retain the recommendation that infants should be breastfed for the first 4-6 months of their lives. The 2008 report does reflect a number of changes as compared with those issued in 2000. Listed below are some of the notable changes.

AAP 2000 Report Recommendations:

- Pregnant women who have risks for allergic diseases should avoid eating peanuts

- Breastfeeding women should avoid peanuts and tree nuts, and should consider avoiding milk, egg and fish.

- Introduce solid foods at 4-6 months; avoid peanuts, nuts and fish until age 3, avoid egg until age 2, avoid milk until age 1.

AAP 2008 Report Recommendations:

- No dietary recommendations are made for pregnant and breastfeeding women.

- Introduce solid foods at 4-6 months; no evidence supports the need to delay the introduction of allergenic foods.

►Can a Food Allergy Be Outgrown?

Peanuts and Tree Nuts: Although a diagnosis of peanut allergy usually indicates a lifelong allergy, there is now evidence that 20% of peanut-allergic children will outgrow their allergy by the age of six years. A study conducted in 2003 found that children who by the age of four have an IgE level to peanut less than 5 kUA/L, will have a 50% chance of passing an oral food challenge to peanut. This study recommends, however, that an oral food challenge to peanut should only be given to individuals who are at least four years of age and who also have an IgE level of 2 kUA/L or less. An oral food challenge should only be done in a clinical setting under the supervision of the child's physician. An important study reported in a 2008 *Journal of Allergy and Clinical Immunology* found that the likelihood of remission of one's peanut allergy can be predicted if there is a low level of IgE antibodies to peanut found during the first two years of a child's life OR if ImmunoCAP blood test results indicate decreasing levels of IgE antibodies to peanut by three years of age. Research data also indicates that if a peanut-allergic individual also has a tree nut and/or a sesame allergy, this will reduce the chances that the peanut allergy will be outgrown. Several research studies have concluded that once a physician has determined that an individual has outgrown his/her peanut allergy, that person should continue to eat peanut products on a regular basis. Data suggests that once outgrown, if peanut is not consumed with some regularity, there is a risk that the allergy will reoccur. The prognosis for outgrowing a tree nut allergy is similar to that of peanut allergy; only a small percentage (9%) will outgrow their nut allergy. Lastly, the likelihood of outgrowing a tree nut allergy is greatly reduced if the person is allergic to more than one tree nut.

Milk: It appears that milk allergy may not be outgrown as early in life as once thought. It was once believed that the majority of children would outgrow their milk allergy somewhere between the ages of three to six years old. In a 2007 study, however, it was determined that 79% of individuals will outgrow their milk allergy by the age of sixteen.

Eggs: Statistics show that 1-2% of young children will have an egg allergy. Although it was once generally accepted that most children would outgrow their egg allergy by the age of five or six, more recent data indicates that 68% of children will outgrow their egg allergy by the time they reach sixteen years old.

Fish and Shellfish: Allergies to these two foods are currently considered to be lifelong. Data suggests that only 2-5% of children will outgrow a fish or shellfish allergy.

Wheat: Wheat allergy is typically outgrown by the time a child reaches five years of age, and is not found in most adults.

Soy: It is generally thought that a soy allergy will usually be outgrown sometime during early childhood. Results of a study conducted in 2010 which looked at the natural history of soy allergy found that 50% of the children in the study outgrew their soy allergy by the age of seven. This study also found that for children with allergy to both soy and lentils, it may take more time for them to outgrow their soy allergy.

►Current Research for the Treatment of Food Allergies!

The information provided below includes examples of some of the research currently being investigated to treat food allergy.

Oral Immunotherapy: Oral immunotherapy is currently being investigated by researchers as a treatment method to desensitize a person to his food allergen. This type of therapy involves having the allergic individual ingest very small amounts of the food to which he is allergic, over a certain period of time. Results of oral immunotherapy studies for milk allergy have been encouraging. Two separate studies conducted in 2008 found that for some individuals with severe milk allergy, this type of treatment resulted in an improvement in the ability to tolerate milk. Another study looking at oral immunotherapy for peanut allergy was reported in a 2009 *Journal of Allergy and Clinical Immunology*. Results of this study found that 27 out of 29 subjects who completed the treatment were able to ingest 3.9 grams of peanut protein during an oral food challenge. Allergic symptoms experienced during oral immunotherapy treatment were found to be mild, and were successfully resolved by using antihistamines.

The role of oral immunotherapy in desensitizing an individual to his food allergen seems to hold promise. Further research is needed in order to determine the overall safety of this type of treatment approach, however. In addition, data gathered from subsequent studies will help to clarify whether the results of oral immunotherapy may be considered long term or are just a temporary response to treatment. *Because of the potential risks, oral immunotherapy is presently considered a research procedure and is not yet approved as treatment. It should only be conducted in a setting under the direction and supervision of the physicians and scientists involved in the study. This is the* **only** *way that the care and safety of the participants can be properly addressed.*

Food Allergy Herbal Formula-2 (FAHF-2): A 2009 study was conducted to determine if herbal formula FAHF-2 would be effective in protecting peanut-allergic mice from anaphylaxis after treatment had been completed. It also sought to determine the long-term effects of this treatment. The resulting data showed that mice involved in this study were protected from the symptoms of anaphylaxis for more than six months after the seven week-long treatment was discontinued. Mice in this study also continued to have reduced peanut-specific IgE levels. What is particularly encouraging about this study is that the FAFH-2 formula did not cause a general immune system response; only the production of IgE antibodies to peanut was suppressed, leaving the rest of the immune system to function normally, as it should. Currently, FAFH-2 is being tested by the U.S. Food and Drug Administration in patients with food allergy.

Our understanding of food allergies and allergic diseases is changing based on the results of current and future research. Because information on this health issue is continually being updated, recommendations regarding how to avoid and treat food allergies are invariably changing, also. Therefore, it is important for pregnant and breastfeeding women, and parents of children with food allergies, to seek the advice and guidance of their doctors, with the understanding that recommendations are offered based on current knowledge.

Conclusion

It should be clear that food allergies present a health issue which must be better understood and better managed. The National Institute of Health's expert panel on food allergy research stated in their 2006 report that " . . . food allergy has emerged as an important public health problem based on its increasing prevalence, persistence throughout life for those who are sensitized to the foods most likely to cause severe reactions (peanut and tree nut), the potential for fatal reactions, and lack of preventive treatment other than food avoidance." In Chapter Two, the growing issue of food allergies and their impact on the school environment will be explored. Guidance regarding realistic and practical recommendations for their management at school will be discussed.

SUPPLEMENTAL MATERIALS

FOOD ALLERGIES: KEY POINTS

- A true food allergy involves an abnormal response of the immune system and causes the body to produce IgE antibodies to a particular food protein. The most severe form of this reaction is called **anaphylaxis.**

- If not treated promptly, anaphylaxis may result in death.

- Food-induced anaphylaxis accounts for approximately 150-200 deaths per year.

- Symptoms of an allergic reaction can be caused by as little as 2 milligrams (1/250th of a peanut) of a peanut, for example. The amount of allergen needed to cause a reaction varies from person to person.

- A food *intolerance*, which does not involve the body's immune system, should **not** be confused with a true food *allergy*.

- Most food allergic reactions occur from eating an unexpected or hidden ingredient, or unknowingly ingesting the allergen from cross-contamination.

- Symptoms of a reaction, such as vomiting, hives or respiratory distress, may vary from person to person.

- Some individuals may develop symptoms of an allergic reaction when the allergen comes in contact with their skin (tactile) OR from inhaling airborne particles of the food protein.

- There is no way to predict how an allergic reaction will develop. Symptoms may progress from mild to severe in several minutes.

- Children are the largest group of the population, (~8%), affected by food allergies.

- Asthma is a risk factor for fatal anaphylaxis in food-allergic children.

- The incidence of peanut allergy in the U.S. has tripled since 1997.

- A *New England Journal of Medicine* study found that **4 out of 6 fatalities** from a food allergic reaction **OCCURRED AT SCHOOL**.

AVOIDANCE is the **ONLY** way to prevent accidental ingestion and a possible life-threatening reaction.

NOTE: Children with documented, life-threatening food allergies may be considered for protection under both state and federal disability laws.

Anaphylaxis Diagnostic Criteria

"Anaphylaxis is a serious allergic reaction that is rapid in onset and may cause death."

Anaphylaxis is highly likely to occur when any one of the following 3 criteria are met:

1. SKIN SYMPTOMS OR SWOLLEN LIPS AND EITHER:
   a. DIFFICULTY BREATHING **OR**
   b. REDUCED BLOOD PRESSURE

2. AN INDIVIDUAL HAD EXPOSURE TO A "SUSPECTED ALLERGEN"
   AND 2 OR MORE OF THE FOLLOWING OCCUR:
   a. SKIN SYMPTOMS OR SWOLLEN LIPS OR TONGUE
   b. DIFFICULTY BREATHING
   c. REDUCED BLOOD PRESSURE
   d. GASTRO-INTESTINAL SYMPTOMS SUCH AS VOMITTING, DIARRHEA OR CRAMPING

3. AN INDIVIDUAL HAS HAD EXPOSURE TO A "KNOWN ALLERGEN"
   AND EXPERIENCES:
   a. REDUCED BLOOD PRESSURE

(Symptoms may occur within minutes to hours after exposure to the allergen.)

Epinephrine should be given immediately when the above criteria are met _or_ for an individual with a history of life-threatening reactions who has had exposure to an allergen and begins to have symptoms quickly, even if they are mild.

Source: Adapted from: 2nd NIAID/FAAN Anaphylaxis Symposium, 7/2005

ALLERGENS AS HIDDEN INGREDIENTS IN FOODS

__MILK__ may be found in the following products: sherbet, hot dogs, deli meats, yogurt, quick breads, gravies, dips, cake mixes, non-dairy creamers, canned tuna fish, ham, popsicles, crackers, baby crackers, bread, rolls, Tostito chips® (lime), Cheetos®, pretzels, cookies, chocolate, cereals, microwave popcorn

"K", "U", "Circle U" = __KOSHER__ label which means that a food has been certified by a Rabbi as meeting the Jewish standard for dietary restrictions of milk, meat, and shellfish.

"K-D", "D", or "DE" = presence of milk protein or foods that were processed on equipment also used for milk products.

*Individuals with a dairy allergy should avoid eating foods which have any of these symbols.

"PAREVE" = foods that *usually* do not contain dairy products or meat products.

__EGGS__ may be found in the following products: glaze on baked goods, mayonnaise, pasta, custard bases to ice cream, baked goods, pancakes, waffles, candy, jelly beans, fried foods from vendors who use the same vat for egg-battered foods.

__PEANUTS__ may be found in the following products: chili, brown gravy, spaghetti sauce, egg rolls, hot cocoa, candy, gourmet popcorn, granola bars, pesto sauce, instant rice mixes, ice cream, Good Humor™ ice cream, chocolates (cross-contamination), M&Ms®,

brownie mix, barbecue sauce, cereals, jelly beans (especially gourmet brands), snack size chips & cookies, gummy bears, and mandelonas (peanuts soaked in almond flavoring).

TREE NUTS may be found in the following products: ice cream, yogurt, candies, cookies, breads, muffins, baked goods, sauces, salad dressings, pie crusts, barbecue sauce, granola bars, pesto, marzipan, cake mixes, brownie mixes, cereals, trail & snack mixes, snack size chips & cookies

SEAFOOD may be found in the following products: caesar salad, Worcestershire sauce, salad dressing, bouillabaisse, surimi (imitation crabmeat)

Note: not all brands of the foods on this list will contain these allergens. This is not a complete list of foods containing allergens.

FOODS THAT ARE *NOT* NUTS
nutmeg: seed from tropical tree   water chestnut: edible plant root

MANUFACTURER DISCLAIMER STATEMENTS

- may contain . . . .

- made on shared equipment with . . . .

- processed in the same plant as . . . .

Copyright © 2012 Educating for Food Allergies, LLC

"Any commitment is only as good as the most knowledgeable, determined, and vigorous person on it. There must be somebody who provides the flame."

Lady Bird Johnson

CHAPTER TWO

GOING TO SCHOOL WITH FOOD ALLERGIES: A 3-STEP PLAN FOR FOOD ALLERGY MANAGEMENT

Background

Most parents, when sending their child off to school, are typically interested in investigating such things as class size, teacher-student ratio, quality of curriculum, etc. Parents of children with food allergies, however, although they may share these same concerns, must also take into consideration several other critical factors when investigating the merits of a potential school for their child to attend. They need to make certain that the school environment is not only educationally sound, but will also provide a safe environment for their child. For parents who are sending their child with food allergies off to school for the first time, this can be a particularly difficult and frightening prospect.

School staff must also address these same concerns as they contemplate the entry of a student with food allergies. Meeting the special needs of a student with food allergies is a multi-faceted and often time-consuming task. It is, however, the school's responsibility to look for ways in which to keep their student population safe, including those children with life-threatening food allergies, while also promoting an atmosphere which allows the students to thrive in all aspects of their education. It is a fair expectation on the part of all parents that schools will be prepared and knowledgeable to meet this obligation. Every child is entitled to feel safe at school and be fully engaged in all of the activities available to them. The information included in this chapter demonstrates the challenge this concept presents, and highlights practical recommendations for developing, implementing and maintaining a comprehensive food allergy management plan intended to enhance the safety of students with food allergies.

Report of EpiPen® Administration at School, MA Department of Public Health

Chapter One presents an overwhelming abundance of evidence which allows us to conclude that: 1.) the number of school-aged children with food allergies is significantly high and increasing, 2.) the symptoms of an allergic reaction and anaphylaxis can be profoundly devastating, and 3.) the school environment presents a real risk to the safety of students with food allergies. Data suggests that it is likely a student with a food allergy will, at some point, experience a food-related allergic reaction at school. Support for this disturbing conclusion may be found in the results of a important initiative begun by the Massachusetts Department of Public Health (MA DPH), School Health Unit, during the school calendar year 2003-2004. A Massachusetts state regulation, 105 CMR 210, has mandated since November, 2003, that schools must file a report with the MA DPH whenever epinephrine has been administered. Since 2003, the MA DPH has annually collected and analyzed data reported to them by both public and private schools across the state of Massachusetts regarding their use of epinephrine for the treatment of allergic reactions during the school day (reports are titled: Data Health Brief: Epinephrine Administration in Schools).

Analysis of the data from the academic years 2003-2004 to 2009-2010 demonstrates that annually, there have been between 133 and 225 administrations of epinephrine during the school day reported, resulting in a seven year cumulative total of 1,118 administrations of this lifesaving medication. Although each year there has been a small percentage of adult staff treated with epinephrine, the overwhelming majority of individuals who have required this treatment are children between the ages of five and eighteen. Although epinephrine was used to treat allergic reactions to such things as food, bees, latex and medications, food appears to have consistently provided the largest percentage of instances where epinephrine was required. The data also reveals that while symptoms of allergic reactions occurred most frequently in the classroom, no area of the school environment has been without risk. Students experienced symptoms of an allergic reaction in virtually all areas of the campus, including in the cafeteria, on the playground and on the bus. One surprising and equally alarming statistic is that each year, between 20-27% of individuals who have needed epinephrine to treat anaphylaxis are individuals not previously identified to school staff as having an allergic condition.

The importance of these annual reports for Massachusetts schools cannot be overstated. If these reports in any way reflect similar occurrences in other states where large numbers of students are experiencing allergic reactions which require treatment with epinephrine, then their relevance becomes even more significant. The hard data and analysis provided by the MA DPH in these reports should serve as a tool to aid all individuals interested in understanding the epidemiology of epinephrine administration at school. In addition, the resulting information may greatly contribute to a better understanding of the risks food allergies present for children who have this health condition, and indicate more productive ways to reduce exposure to allergens at school so that the incidence and trauma of anaphylaxis can be significantly reduced.

The MA DPH's annual report documenting the epidemiology of epinephrine administration for the treatment of allergic reactions in Massachusetts schools, when combined with the results of studies shared in the previous chapter, provide strong and clear evidence that children with food allergies are continuing to be exposed to their allergens at school and are experiencing anaphylactic reactions as a result. Although the standard treatment for anaphylaxis is epinephrine, it can not always be counted on with absolute certainty. Dr. Hugh Sampson, a leading researcher in the area of food allergies, and an allergist at Mount Sinai Hospital in New York, reported that 7%-10% of individuals died from food-induced anaphylaxis despite prompt treatment with epinephrine. The results of this study should make clear the fact that treatment with epinephrine cannot be relied upon as the primary or sole focus for food allergy management at school.

Study on Current School Food Allergy Management Deficiencies

Michael Young, M.D., allergist and author of *The Peanut Allergy Answer Book, Second Edition,* Anne Munoz-Furlong, founder of The Food Allergy and Anaphylaxis Network and Scott Sicherer, M.D., allergist and author of *Understanding and Managing Your Child's Food Allergies*, are three individuals who have spent a great deal of their lives dedicated to the issue of food allergies. They recently joined forces in an effort to evaluate current food allergy management practices at school. As a result of this initiative, their analysis of data and information collected was reported in 2009 in the *Journal of Allergy and Clinical Immunology*. Their study revealed two main deficiencies in food allergy and anaphylaxis management at school:

1.) Food allergy management plans being used are inadequate, and

2.) There is inadequate recognition and treatment of anaphylaxis with epinephrine.

In order for food allergy management plans to be effective, they must be comprehensive. Furthermore, if the ultimate goal of school food allergy management is to prevent allergic reactions from happening, then there is a critical need for schools to incorporate proactive strategies to reduce the likelihood of students from coming into contact with their allergens. Equally important is the need for *all* school staff to be educated in recognizing the symptoms of an allergic reaction, for school staff to be trained to properly administer epinephrine by auto-injector, and for epinephrine to be readily available in the event that an allergic reaction should occur. Based on my personal experience and my professional work with schools and families over the past seventeen years on this issue, I believe that in order to accomplish these important endeavors, an effective food allergy management program at school should encompass three main goals:

STEP ONE: Avoidance: procedures must be put into place which reduce the risk of children with food allergies from coming into contact with their allergen(s),

STEP TWO: Education: procedures must be put into place which educate the entire school community in understanding food allergies and ways to prevent allergic reactions,

STEP THREE: Response: procedures must be put into place which allow for the prompt response and treatment of an allergic reaction.

It is important for parents and schools to realize that this challenge is not insurmountable and that there are tangible steps which can be taken to achieve these three goals.

STEP ONE: AVOIDANCE

The fundamental premise for managing an effective food allergy management program is "avoidance". Stated simply, this refers to procedures utilized at school which are intended to reduce students' chances of being exposed to their allergens. The critical role of this strategy is emphasized by Dr. Hugh Sampson when he says, "The life-threatening nature of anaphylaxis makes prevention the cornerstone of therapy". Direct support of this approach may be found in a position statement issued by The American Academy of Allergy, Asthma and Immunology (AAAAI) in 1998 entitled, *"Anaphylaxis in Schools and Other Childcare Settings"*. It states:

"The most important aspect of the management of patients with life-threatening allergies is avoidance . . . Furthermore, school personnel should work in partnership with the parents to develop strategies for avoiding a reaction while allowing the student to participate fully in all activities."

There are several national organizations, such as the National Association of School Nurses, the National Association of Elementary School Principals, the National Association of Secondary School Principals, the National School Board Association, along with the Food Allergy and Anaphylaxis Network, who have joined together to develop a similar position statement on managing food allergies at school. These organizations, in their collective effort, promote the need for avoidance practices as well as the need for all school staff to be trained and knowledgeable about food allergy issues. (See Supplemental Materials at end of chapter.)

The Massachusetts Department of Education, with their 2002 publication entitled, "Managing Life Threatening Food Allergies in Schools", was the first state in the nation to develop school food allergy management guidelines. The clear message delivered in this major work is that "total avoidance of the substance to which the student is allergic is the only means to prevent food allergy reactions." In recent years, several other states have written similar guidelines which echo this same premise in an effort to assist school staff in their food allergy management efforts.

How do you accomplish the goal of "avoidance?"

A plan for the "avoidance" of a student's allergens may be accomplished by utilizing one of two strategies:

1. An Individual Healthcare Plan (IHP)

   OR

2. A 504 Plan (children with documented life-threatening food allergies are eligible for protection under Section 504 of the Rehabilitation Act of 1973. Please refer to Chapter 4 for more information on 504 Plans).

Individual Healthcare Plans (IHP)

We will first look at the IHP as a means of food allergy management at school. Any child with a food allergy should have a thorough IHP in place at school for the prevention of food-allergic reactions. This strategy and approach is supported and stressed in the Massachusetts Department of Education's written guidelines on school food allergy management referenced earlier in this chapter. Having worked with both schools and families in this field for many years, I cannot stress enough how important the development of an IHP is as the most productive *and* proactive means to accomplish the critical goal of reducing the risk of an allergic reaction from occurring at school.

What is an IHP?

An IHP is a written healthcare plan intended to manage a student's food allergies. It establishes safe practices and procedures for the student and focuses on prevention as its primary strategy. As represented in its title, an Individual Healthcare Plan must be developed for an *individual* student, in order to meet the needs of *that* student. It is important for this healthcare plan to be as comprehensive as possible by addressing 1.) all aspects of the school environment and 2.) all aspects of the school day, including before, during and after school hours when school-sponsored events take place.

Attention must be focused on each area within the school environment where the student will travel, including those found both in and outside of the school building itself. In other words, procedures which reduce the student's risk of exposure to his/her food allergens need to be put into place not only in the classroom and cafeteria, but also for activities such as gym, art, computer class, recess and field trips. Furthermore, avoidance procedures within the student's IHP must also address any and all activities planned and sponsored by the school, including those that are scheduled to take place before or after normal school hours. This would include then, before or after school music or sports practices, or a school-sponsored dance or event, for example. Activities that take place at school, but are not school-sponsored events, such as Boy or Girl Scout meetings or Little League practice, are not the responsibility of the school. Procedures meant to address the safety of the participating students must be arranged by those organizations themselves, in conjunction with the students' parents.

It is important to think of planning an IHP as a process that requires ongoing coordination between the school and the parents of the food-allergic student. The first step would be for the parents to notify the school of their child's food allergies well before the first day of school. Whenever information of particular importance is communicated to school officials, it is highly recommended that it always be done in writing, in the form of a letter or email, for example. In this case, parents should compose a letter or email addressed to the school nurse that indicates that their child has food allergies, and request that a meeting be scheduled as soon as possible. The letter should indicate that the purpose of this meeting is to 1.) inform the nurse and school of their child's health and any related concerns, 2.) determine what procedures are currently in place at the school to manage food allergies, and 3.) begin the process of developing specific procedures within an individual healthcare plan which meet the individual needs of their child. In instances where there is not a school nurse on staff, it is recommended that the letter be addressed to the attention of the principal or head of school.

It is important to recognize that information sometimes gets misplaced or becomes stagnant on what may be a lengthy "to do" list. If extensive time has passed without receiving a response from a school official, then it is advisable for the parent to make continued attempts to reach school personnel on this matter until a connection has been made.

Who Develops the IHP?

Once a child with life-threatening food allergies has been identified to the school, it is the responsibility of the school nurse, (or school administrator if there is not a nurse), to respond to this information and schedule a meeting with the family. It is optimal for this meeting to take place before the first day of school. The school nurse is the key player in coordinating and overseeing a child's health issues at school. As such, the school nurse has the responsibility of being the "initiator" of the Individualized Healthcare Plan and the "implementer" of its plan for avoidance practices and emergency response. The school nurse may be viewed as the "case manager" for coordinating and overseeing the child's care and should serve as the point of contact at school for all health-related questions. Therefore, the nurse needs to make every effort to connect with the parents of the food-allergic student. This often requires perseverance and the utilization of all forms of communication possible: in-person meetings, the telephone and/or email, for example. In other words, whatever is effective! A comprehensive IHP that serves as a productive tool in keeping a student with life-threatening food allergies safe makes this level of effort appropriate and worthwhile.

During the first scheduled meeting it is important for both the nurse and the parents to establish a good working relationship which is viewed by all as a true partnership. It is the parent's responsibility to bring copies of all medical documentation of their child's allergies and any related health issues required by the school. This would be the time for parents to discuss their child's allergies and level of sensitivity, the circumstances of prior allergic reactions, symptoms that their child typically presents, and other health considerations such as asthma and eczema. Providing information about their child's personality can also be enormously helpful. This could assist not only in better decision-making regarding teacher assignments, but would also help school staff to have a clearer understanding of the child and how he or she may react to various scenarios as they relate to having a food allergy. A parent's insight and experience should never be underestimated and may be the source of invaluable information at this meeting.

It is the school nurse's responsibility to provide information about procedures currently being utilized at the school to manage food allergies, such as in the classroom, cafeteria, at recess, on field trips and for bus transportation. This should include sharing with the parents which staff members are trained to administer the epinephrine by auto-injector and where this life-saving medicine is kept. Once information has been shared, and in a cooperative spirit, the parents and school nurse should begin the process of developing a comprehensive individual healthcare plan intended to reduce the risk of the student from allergen exposure. This process may require more than one meeting; adequate time should be planned to allow for the thoughtful development of the student's IHP. When the process is completed, both the school nurse and the parents should feel with confidence, that the IHP is reasonable and meets the student's needs.

Once all aspects of the IHP have been developed and agreed upon by both the parents and nurse, it should be put *in writing*. No matter how competent we are, it is unrealistic to believe that strategies devised and decisions made of such importance will be remembered in the detail that is required, especially with the passage of time, if they are not put down on paper. Putting this document in writing allows all who have a vested interest in its content to refer back to it whenever questions arise. Once the IHP is finalized and in written form, the best practice would be for the parents and nurse to sign and date it. These signatures demonstrate the good faith and intent of both parties to uphold their responsibilities as they pertain to the student's IHP.

The process of developing and implementing the procedures within an IHP requires a multi-disciplinary approach. Consequently, the next step would be for the nurse to schedule a meeting with all school staff who will have direct contact with the student, along with the student's parents. This collection of school personnel is sometimes referred to as the "core team". School personnel who should be included in this meeting are typically the child's classroom teacher, specialist teachers, such as art, music, gym, librarian, computer, and the directors of food service and bus transportation. Once again, timing is important. Whenever possible, this meeting should be scheduled to take place prior to the start of the school year so that there is sufficient time to review the content of the IHP and discuss staff's role in its implementation. Having the parents at this meeting is important because inevitably staff members will have questions or need clarifications that are best answered by the student's parents. Developing an IHP requires cooperation, advance planning, the allocation of sufficient time to plan and patience among everyone. Each individual involved will have an important and specific role in helping to insure the success of efforts being made to manage a student's food allergies.

FOOD ALLERGIES: A SCHOOL NURSE PERSPECTIVE

Partnerships are so important when it comes to food allergies. As a school nurse with over 30 years experience, I tell parents that I will not guarantee them or their child a peanut or nut free school. However, I will work with them to make the school environment as safe as possible for their child. The old quote "It takes a village" is so true when it comes to food allergies. Parents, physicians, school staff and students working together are an important and great partnership.

School nurses need to meet with the parents and usually the day of registration is not enough time. They must choose a comfortable time for both the parents and nurse that will allow for all questions to be asked and answered. Because no two situations, parent concerns or children's allergies are the same, plans need to be individualized for each student. A Healthcare Plan should include information and input from the physician, nurse and parent. The nurse needs to know what allergens the child has tested positive for, how did the child react (rash, face swelling, difficulty breathing, vomiting, diarrhea, etc.). What did the child say: "my mouth feels funny", "my throat is itchy", or "I think I am going to die". I can't stress enough how each description and reaction can be different.

The nurse should go over the school policy and procedures on food allergies, explaining training of staff, designation of a food allergy classroom, hand washing, area for snack and lunch, if necessary, school parties, who reads labels, child-specific extra snacks, plans for field trips, daily transportation and most importantly, the storage of EpiPen®s. Many times this information may need to be repeated and reinforced during the year, as it's a lot to absorb at one time. The training of staff includes administration, classroom teachers, specialists, secretaries, paraprofessionals, cafeteria workers, custodians and bus drivers. If a child will be buying lunch, we need to remind parents to check with the cafeteria staff about ingredients. Don't assume that next week's pizza will be the same. Schools frequently change vendors and the ingredients change, too. Parents need to call and check each time—school staff should welcome the questions and want to help keep the student safe.

Partnerships and flexibility are the key words. Many times we need to be flexible and change a plan to fit a different situation. Together our goal is to keep the student and all children in school safe, healthy and ready to learn.

Judi McAuliffe, RN, NCSN, School Nurse Leader, Pembroke, Massachusetts

How Should an IHP be Formatted?

At this writing, there is no universal form or template for schools to use as an IHP form for their food-allergic students. In fact, there appears to be a lack of forms appropriate for this purpose, in general. As a result, many schools within the same district often utilize different IHP forms for their students with food allergies. Unfortunately, this practice may contribute to a lack of coordination and understanding of IHP content and meaning, between school nurses within the district. Additionally, many schools are using IHP forms that resemble care plans better suited for use in a hospital. Consequently, IHP forms currently in use range from being efficient in their design to woefully inadequate.

It is critical that an IHP form be clear, concise and tailored specifically for use in the school setting. Ideally, it is recommended that this form be comprised of two distinct parts. Part One should cover basic identifying information for the student, such as the student's name, address, telephone number, the parent's name(s) and contact information, the school attended, the academic year and the student's grade, and the teacher's name, for example. In addition, this section should indicate medical information, such as the child's allergies and any related health concerns, and the allergist's name and contact information.

Part Two of an IHP should be thought of as the "plan of action" for the student, and should outline, in detail, avoidance procedures to be followed in order for the student to attend school more safely. The format of this section needs to be displayed in a direct and user-friendly manner. It should be formatted to have headings which clearly identify:

1.) Each area of the school in which the student will travel,

2.) Potential risks to the student's safety that exist in each area of the school,

3.) Avoidance procedures meant to reduce each risk,

4.) Each staff member who will be responsible for implementing or overseeing each avoidance procedure.

This may be thought of as the required "recipe of ingredients" needed for an IHP to serve its purpose of enhancing the safety of a child with food allergies at school. Attention must be paid to *all* of the components listed above in order to achieve the goal of preventing the student from experiencing an allergic reaction while at school.

The process of planning avoidance practices for Part Two of the IHP can prove to be overwhelming at times. As stated previously, a universal IHP template which could facilitate this process, currently does not exist. In order to assist school nurses with this important task, my consulting company developed an IHP worksheet that presents an easy to follow, step-by-step format which allows this task to be more easily accomplished. With this worksheet, planning a thorough IHP may proceed in a systematic and organized way. (See IHP and IHP Worksheet Forms at the end of this chapter).

SECTION 504 PLANS

Another way in which to address the needs of a student with life-threatening food allergies is by utilizing a 504 Plan. A 504 Plan is a product of the provisions found in Section 504 of the Rehabilitation Act of 1973 which is a federal law enforced by the U.S. Office of Civil Rights (OCR) within the U.S. Department of Education. This law was enacted to "prohibit discrimination on the basis of disability in education . . . in any program or institution receiving federal funds." Most public schools and many private schools are subject to the requirements of this law because they receive federal funding in one form or another.

ELIGIBILITY

Eligibility for protection under Section 504 requires the student to have a disability that substantially limits one or more life activities. The OCR formally recognizes "allergy" as a "hidden disability", which may be defined as any mental or physical impairment that is not visible to other individuals. The specific criteria which allows someone with a food allergy to be eligible for protection under Section 504 is that the physiological condition of food allergy affects the respiratory, cardiovascular and skin body systems. Therefore, children with physician-documented, life-threatening food allergies may be considered to have a disability under this law, and as such, may be eligible for protection under Section 504. Consequently, a 504 Plan is an appropriate means to manage a student's life threatening food allergy at school.

Schools should have a formal procedure for a child to be considered for protection under Section 504. Anyone familiar with the student, such as the student's parents, the school nurse, the teacher or principal, may request an **evaluation meeting** to be scheduled in order to determine the child's eligibility for protection. This request, which I recommend should always be put in writing, is usually made with the staff member at the school who is assigned Section 504 responsibilities. In some instances, however, it is necessary to contact the 504 Coordinator at the school district level. Once this request has been received, the student's parents should be notified of the meeting date and time.

The individuals present at a Section 504 evaluation meeting are typically the school's 504 Coordinator, the school nurse, the principal, the classroom teacher and the parents of the child being evaluated. It should be noted that although it is not legally required for the parents to be present at this meeting, it is considered the best practice. Additional individuals who have an appropriate reason to attend this meeting may also be included. If a determination is made that the student should receive Section 504 protection, the next step would be for the school nurse to plan a meeting to develop accommodations which address the special healthcare needs of the student. It is also considered best practice for the student's parents to be included in the planning of appropriate accommodations for their child. Section 504 protection means that modifications may need to be made to classroom curriculum and procedures if current procedures are found to put the student's safety at risk.

There is no standard template for 504 Plans, which means that the form used by one school district may be formatted completely differently in another school district. What does appear to be common is the use of forms which more appropriately address a student's physical disabilities and often refer to equipment needed. In addition, the area for accommodations is typically quite limited, and usually does not provide sufficient space to provide a comprehensive list of accommodations necessary to address the management of a student's life threatening food allergies. Because of this, it is an acceptable practice to physically attach a student's IHP to the 504 Plan, and use this as the "accommodations" section for the 504 Plan.

Comparison of an Individualized Healthcare Plan versus a Section 504 Plan

It is important to understand that there are significant similarities and differences between these two management strategies as you evaluate which approach will best meet the needs of the student with food allergies. The major similarity between an IHP and a Section 504 Plan is that either plan should establish written procedures meant to manage a student's food allergies at school. There are, however, several important differences to note between an IHP and a Section 504 Plan. First, because a 504 Plan is a product of a federal law, it is considered a legal document. Consequently, a formalized procedure is followed by school personnel in order to determine both a student's eligibility for protection and the accommodations which will be implemented at school for that student. An IHP, on the other hand, is considered a documented plan of care, and typically involves a much more informal planning process. Second, the school staff member responsible for Section 504 compliance, is the person who organizes and takes the lead role in a Section 504 Plan meeting. This individual is not usually involved at all in planning a student's IHP, but rather it is the school nurse who is in charge. Third, a Section 504 Plan has a formal grievance procedure, which may be pursued by either school personnel or the student's parents, should a dispute develop regarding care for the student which cannot be resolved at the local, district level. Conversely, when an IHP is pursued, there is no formal grievance procedure available for the parents or school staff to follow, should a disagreement occur.

In my experience, utilizing an IHP as a means to manage a student's food allergies at school is an appropriate and good place to start. A Section 504 Plan would be an important management strategy to pursue if disagreements develop between school personnel and the student's parents regarding such things as the nature of a student's accommodations and/or failure of staff to implement healthcare accommodations. Both of these scenarios could result in putting the student's safety at risk. Ultimately, however, either an IHP or a Section 504 Plan, when it is thoughtfully written and carefully implemented, will provide accommodations which will enhance the safety and well-being of the student with food allergies.

(Please refer to Chapter Four for more specific information about 504 Plans and Section 504 of the Rehabilitation Act of 1973.)

FOOD ALLERGEN AVOIDANCE STRATEGIES

A *School-Wide* Peanut/Nut Ban

We know that children with a peanut or tree nut allergy are at a higher risk for having anaphylaxis, and that these two foods are responsible for 90% of fatal food-allergic reactions. Therefore, it is not unusual for questions about banning peanuts and nuts from school to be explored by both parents of peanut-allergic children and their school principals and nurses. It is a question motivated by the desire to keep students with these life threatening food allergies safe from their allergens while at school. The decision of whether to impose a school-wide ban on peanuts and nuts, however, requires careful thought and consideration of a variety of important factors.

First, the task of making a school environment peanut and nut free, and subsequently managing it as such, is not an easy undertaking. Success at achieving this outcome is really dependent upon the cooperation of *every* individual within the school community: school administrators—teachers—auxiliary staff—parents—students. School administrators would need to schedule and provide education to everyone within the school community in order to 1.) facilitate an understanding of food allergies, 2.) explain what will be involved with a school-wide ban, and 3.) convey what responsibilities will be required of each person in order to make the plan work. For instance, if the school cafeteria typically serves items such as peanut butter sandwiches and nut-encrusted ice creams, then the food service director will need to investigate and arrange for food choices that do not include these ingredients. Similarly, *all* parents will need to know specifically what foods are safe to send for snacks and lunch, in addition to understanding what foods must be avoided.

Without a doubt, consideration must be given to determine effective venues in order to communicate this important information to the entire school community. Language used must be clear and leave no room for misinterpretation. Some schools provide essential information in letters, emails and in school handbooks and newsletters. School meetings scheduled at the beginning of the year provide an excellent opportunity to communicate pertinent information, while also allowing for questions to be asked and answered.

Although education is paramount for most people to become "on board" with this goal, there inevitably are some individuals who will balk, either simply because they resist being told what they can and can not do, or because they believe that peanut butter is the only food their child will eat, for example. Consequently, feelings of resentment may develop, which may, in turn, lead to public comments that are negative and perhaps even hostile. This can be an awkward and difficult dynamic for both the school and parents of children with these food allergies to address. It is also possible for a student with a peanut or nut allergy to suffer negative repercussions because of the peanut ban and be made to feel that it is their "fault".

Unfortunately, despite educational efforts, some parents may decide, for whatever reason, not to cooperate with peanut/nut free procedures in effect at their child's school. When peanuts and nuts are sent in to a "peanut/nut free" school, either deliberately or by accident, the actual safety of that environment clearly becomes compromised. The possibility of this scenario gives credence to the notion of a "false sense of security" implicit in a plan for a peanut/ nut free school. To avoid resentment and non-cooperation with these procedures, schools must actively work to foster the understanding and cooperation of everyone. The integrity of a peanut/nut free environment can be maintained only when procedures are in place to continually monitor foods coming into the school, in both classrooms and public areas, to insure they are free of these allergens. In addition, proactive procedures must be in place that address those occasions when unsafe foods may be brought to school. These procedures should include replacing the allergenic food with a safe food, so that the child is not left hungry. Isolating or segregating a child while they eat a contraband food is not a recommended solution to this problem, for the same reasons that children with a food allergy should never be treated this way when they are eating.

Lastly, because we are all human, it is important to understand that mistakes can be made, and allergic reactions may happen. Therefore, it is also critical that staff be educated to recognize the signs of a food-allergic reaction and anaphylaxis, and be trained in the proper response to this medical emergency. Emergency response protocols must be a part of food allergy management, even in a school that has a complete ban on peanuts and nuts.

Achieving a true school-wide ban on peanuts and nuts requires a tremendous amount of time and planning. There are many variables to consider, many hurdles to overcome, and many people whose cooperation must be enlisted. The question of whether to impose such a ban on other student's life-threatening allergies may need to be addressed. That being said, there are schools throughout the United States that have chosen to enforce a peanut/nut free ban on the entire school community. This approach to managing food allergies seems most appropriate in an elementary or lower elementary school, where young children are most likely to touch one another, putting the food-allergic students at most risk for being exposed to their allergens. Schools that impose school-wide peanut/nut bans successfully are the schools that fully understand all that is required to make it work.

Food Allergen-Safe Zones: An Alternative to School-Wide Peanut/Nut Bans

The establishment of allergen-safe zones at school, when carefully managed, is a realistic and viable means to allow for the safe participation of students with food allergies at school. This strategy is more easily established and managed than a school-wide ban, because it involves the cooperation of fewer people day to day. Because of this, it is also more feasible to request the exclusion of other life-threatening food allergens, depending on student needs, on a classroom-specific basis. For example, in a classroom that has a student with life threatening allergies to peanuts, eggs and milk, it would be feasible to request that the twenty-five or so families who have a child in this classroom not send in these foods. On the other hand, making this same request of the entire school community would involve not only the cooperation of the cafeteria staff, but also hundreds of families.

Two areas in which students spend a great deal of time are the classroom and the cafeteria. These are also environments where food is regularly present, whether for the purpose of eating or for use in various projects. Careful consideration of procedures meant to keep a student with food allergies safe must occur in order to establish allergen-free zones that meet this objective.

THE CLASSROOM

Allergen-Free Curriculum

One of the most debated questions, it seems, is whether or not to make the student's classroom a food-allergen free zone. Regardless of whether the student is in elementary school, middle school or high school, the standard should be that his/her food allergens will not be used in the curriculum, such as for art, science or cooking projects. To do so would put that student's health and safety at risk. To suggest the child not participate in the activity, or to send the student off to another location, such as the library or health office during the project, are simply not options because such practices would be considered discriminatory. It is a reasonable expectation that the teacher, when health considerations dictate such actions, modify the curriculum plan to allow for the safe participation of *all* their students. If Plan A involves an experiment with raw eggs, for example, and there is a student with an egg allergy in the class, then the teacher needs to utilize Plan B, which uses an alternative, and safe product for the experiment. This safe product should be used for all the students in the class in order to reduce the risk of exposure through skin contact or cross-contamination. Advance planning and consultation with the school nurse and the student's parents, or with the student when age appropriate, such as in the upper grades, is usually all that is required to allow for full participation by *all* students in the class.

What Happened: A middle school student with several food allergies arrived for French class and, along with the other students in the class, was told that they would be cooking that day. When the food-allergic student asked the teacher if any of his allergens would be involved, she replied that she didn't know, and that there was no way to check because she had already discarded some food containers. The student expressed concern over this situation, and the teacher responded by telling him he needed to go to the library during class, and miss the lesson.

What Should Have Happened: Advance planning and communication. Had the teacher checked with the school nurse, the student's parents and/or the student himself prior to the day this activity was to take place, safe food items could easily have been selected and the student would have been able to participate in the lesson.

You Should Know: The teacher may have thought her actions were appropriate, however segregating or isolating a student is considered discriminatory under Section 504 of the Rehabilitation Act of 1973. If a teacher plans an activity believed to have sound educational value for the class, then *all* the students in the class are entitled to benefit from the program.

ALLERGEN-SAFE FOOD FOR CONSUMPTION

Food for consumption in the classroom is another concern for students with a food allergy, particularly for children in the lower elementary grades. It should be understood that successfully avoiding an allergic reaction requires more than teaching a child to understand that they must not eat the offending food. A recent study reported in a 2009 *Journal of Allergy and Clinical Immunology* which evaluated food allergy management procedures, stressed that it is not unusual for young children to touch each other, and each other's food. These common behaviors may, in turn, lead to the student's exposure to their food allergens through either skin contact or cross-contamination. Because many young children put their hands and fingers in their mouths, the study points out that these types of allergen exposures could lead to their ingestion and result in the possibility of a severe allergic reaction. Cheese powder from snack foods such as Cheetos® and Doritos®, for example, may often be found on a person's fingertips after the snack has been eaten. Consequently foods like these pose a serious risk for students with a milk allergy.

Peanut butter is another particularly sticky substance which is easily transferred from one surface to another. Statistics which demonstrate the significantly high number of fatalities caused by peanuts and nuts have undoubtedly contributed to the fact that many classrooms for younger children are being designated as peanut and nut free. In determining if a student's allergen(s) should be eliminated from the classroom, a realistic assessment of the likelihood of the student coming into contact with the allergen must be evaluated. If there is a possibility of allergen exposure, then opting for a classroom safe from a student's allergens is optimal for the student's safety and wellbeing.

No Food Sharing Rules

Implementing a "**no food sharing**" rule is also an important strategy to reduce the chance of accidental ingestion. When this rule is followed, some parents of food-allergic children choose to allow foods that contain advisory warning labels, such as "Made on shared equipment with . . ." in the class, as long as their child understands not to eat these foods. For foods that list "peanut oil" as one of the ingredients, it is interesting to note that most peanut oils manufactured in the United States have been hot-pressed and are therefore highly refined. This process denatures the peanut protein and renders the peanut oil incapable of causing an allergic reaction. The exception to this is gourmet peanut oils, which are typically cold-pressed and therefore still contain peanut protein that could cause an allergic reaction if ingested. It is not always clear on the label whether or not the peanut oil has been cold or hot-pressed. Ultimately, the parents of the child with food allergies must evaluate whether foods containing peanut oil may be allowed in the classroom.

Safe Foods for Snacks and Celebrations

Food for Safe Snacks. Establishing a **safe snack program** is an effective way to prevent the ingestion of food allergens in the classroom. A recommended procedure would be for the parents of the food-allergic child to always provide a safe snack for their child. All other children would bring in their own snack based on a *classroom-specific list of safe snacks* provided by the parent of the child with food allergies. If there is more than one child in the class with food allergies, then it is crucial that the list of safe snacks reflects a coordinated effort between each of the food-allergic children's parents. This will help to insure that all snacks entering the classroom contain only safe ingredients for all of the students in the class. This list should include brand names and the request that ingredients be read by an adult staff member each and every time a product will be sent into the classroom. The food sent into the classroom should be in its original packaging and have visible ingredient labels. Once again, a "no food sharing" rule for the student in the classroom who has the allergy should be followed whenever food is eaten. Hand washing and table surface cleaning practices should also be established and carefully followed.

It is possible that on occasion, a snack containing the student's allergens may be accidentally sent into the classroom. For this reason, the parent of the food-allergic student should maintain a supply of safe snacks in the classroom. The unsafe snack should be put back into the student's backpack for them to bring back home, and the child should be given a safe snack to eat. The details of this procedure and the reasons behind it should be understood by the parents of all children in the class.

Food for Birthday and Holiday Celebrations. It is recommended that the parents of the child with food allergies keep "special" safe snacks at school for their child to eat whenever there is a birthday, holiday or celebration. Non-perishable foods may be kept in a container in the classroom for this purpose. For foods that need to be kept refrigerated or frozen, such as ice cream cups or popsicles, most cafeteria directors are willing to dedicate a small area in the kitchen's refrigerator or freezer to store these items. A classroom-specific list of safe foods and brands for "special" occasions should be developed by the parents of the food-allergic child (or children) and made available to parents of the other children in the class. This allows food consumed in the classroom for celebrations to be special *and* safe regarding cross-contamination issues. As a courtesy, a suggestion would be for the parent of the birthday child to call the parents of the child with food allergies to inform them of the date of the birthday, and to let them know what treat they plan to bring to class. In this way, the parent of the food-allergic child can make arrangements to coordinate a similar treat for their child. This would require solicitation of the food-allergic parents' permission to share their phone number with the other parents in their child's class.

An alternative approach to insure that all foods entering the classroom are safe would be for the parent of the child with food allergies to take responsibility for purchasing *all* snacks, birthday and holiday treats for the entire class. In this scenario, the parents of all classmates would contribute an agreed-upon dollar amount to a fund established for this purpose. These safe snacks would be kept in a large container in the classroom, and replenished as needed. Although this option seems labor intensive for the parent of the food-allergic child, it provides the greatest level of safety for the food-allergic child. Feedback from teachers, parents of the child with food allergies, and parents of the other classmates who have used this procedure, have been overwhelmingly positive. Teachers find that children seem to look forward to snack time, classmates' parents seem to enjoy the freedom of not having to send in a snack, and the parents of the food-allergic child breathe a little easier knowing their child is eating safe foods while at school. For either approach utilized for holidays and celebrations, hand washing and table surface cleaning practices should be a part of the plan.

When Allergens are Allowed for Consumption

For situations in which food allergens are allowed in the classroom during snack and holiday/birthday celebrations, it is recommended that the food-allergic student be assigned to an allergen-free table when these foods are eaten. It should be recognized that this approach does put the student with food allergies at a higher risk for being exposed to their allergens and experiencing an allergic reaction. Therefore, **hand washing** and **table surface washing** practices become extremely paramount in eliminating the transference of food allergens. Good old-fashioned soap and water and commercial wipes have proven to be effective in removing food allergens from the hands, however waterless hand sanitizers, such as Purell®, are not productive in removing food protein. In classes where food allergens are allowed, it is also important that the teacher monitor the students to ensure that food is not being shared, and that strict cleaning procedures are being followed. It is also reasonable to request cooperation on the part of the other parents to reduce the number of foods sent into the classroom that contain the student's allergens. When food allergens are allowed in the classroom, it is important that the child with food allergies understands that only food brought from home may be eaten. Another suggested safety precaution in these classrooms would be for food-allergic children to put a placemat dedicated for their use, or even a napkin, down on the desk before they eat, as added protection. Please refer to "Food-Free Birthday Celebrations" in Supplemental Materials located at the end of this chapter.

Further considerations for planning safe procedures in the classroom:

- **Epinephrine by auto-injector**: Advance planning for the storage of the EpiPen® and the Emergency Treatment Plan. This lifesaving medicine should be maintained in the classroom (in addition to having another EpiPen® kept in the Health Room with the school nurse) and must be kept in a safe location where it can be accessed quickly. Life-saving medication such as epinephrine by auto-injector should never be kept under lock and key during the school day.

- Examination of classroom materials that may contain hidden allergens:

    — empty peanut butter jars or yogurt cups used as containers for manipulatives and writing implements, for example.

    — soaps, which may contain nut or seed oils.

    — pet, bird and fish food, which may contain fish products, milk products, peanut/nut products and wheat products.

— Rubber Cement, which contains natural latex (for latex allergies).

- Planning for cooking and science activities, to ensure no allergens will be used.

- Implementing hand washing practices (recommended for all students in the class, at start of day, after snack and after lunch, especially for preschool and elementary).

- Regard for "High Risk" times, to ensure safe protocols are being practiced. High risk times are defined as those times during which the usual routine is interrupted or different. Examples would be:

— substitute teachers: they must be alerted to procedures practiced in the allergen-free room. Meeting with the school nurse prior to assuming responsibility for the class is highly recommended.

— field trips require that: 1.) the classroom teacher gives advance notice of date of the trip to the school nurse *and* the parents of the child with food allergies, 2.) arrangements are made for all emergency medicines, such as the EpiPen®, the written treatment plan, and an EpiPen®-trained adult to be present on the trip, 3.) there is a reliable form of communication, such as a cell phone, in case of an emergency, 4.) there is knowledge of the nearest hospital, and 5.) plans are made for food allergen avoidance, if food will be consumed on the trip.

— fire drills: procedures must be planned to ensure the student's EpiPen® will be readily accessible.

— "special" programs: events such as Field Day, school dances, band/orchestra concerts and sporting events must be planned to allow for the safe participation of the student with food allergies.

- Peer/parent education is a wonderful way to foster an understanding and acceptance of classroom protocols and procedures. In support of this, allergist Dr. Michael Young states in his *Peanut Allergy Answer Book* that " . . . education of the child's classmates and their families is just as important as the education of the school and its staff."

- The allergen-free classroom should not be used before or after school by other organizations for their meetings or events (*e.g.* Scouts), unless they abide by the food allergy management protocols in place. Procedures should be put into place to ensure this. Some schools have a representative of the organization read and sign a contract agreeing to follow the rules for classroom use.

THE CAFETERIA

Eating lunch in the cafeteria is a social time and allows students the ability to develop appropriate interactions with their peers. Whenever food is eaten, however, there is an increased risk for allergen exposure and subsequently, an allergic reaction and anaphylaxis. The planning of safe procedures in the cafeteria is critical for the physical safety and the emotional well-being of students with food allergies. More and more schools are reducing or eliminating the sale of peanut butter and jelly sandwiches in an effort to reduce the amount of peanut butter present in the school environment. Some schools are significantly reducing or eliminating ice creams and snacks sold that contain peanuts and nuts. Many schools are also requiring that items which will be sold during PTO bake sales must be individually wrapped before they are brought into the cafeteria. All of these efforts demonstrate an understanding of the serious issue food allergies present, and reflect the school's support of efforts intended to help keep students with food allergies safe within the school community.

Epinephrine

In addition to the strong recommendation that a student's EpiPen® be kept in the classroom and also in the nurse's office, it is highly recommended that an additional EpiPen® and the student's Emergency Treatment Plan be kept in a safe place in the cafeteria. These items should be visible only to food service staff, and not other students. (Note: the Emergency Treatment Plan is discussed in detail later in this chapter under "Step Three—Response". Confidentiality issues covered by the Family Education Rights and Privacy Act (FERPA) are discussed in Chapter Four.)

Food Handling Practices

All Food Service personnel should be trained in general food allergy education. This should include knowledge of common food allergen terminology and an understanding of the serious risk cross-contamination issues present to students with food allergies who buy their lunch. Specific procedures intended to avoid this risk must be implemented regarding food preparation, food serving, and thorough cleaning of pots, pans, utensils and countertops. An added safety precaution would be for schools that serve peanut butter and jelly sandwiches to consider pre-making and wrapping these sandwiches early in the day. Any utensils used in the making of these sandwiches should be put immediately in the dishwasher after use. Latex gloves should not be used in order to accommodate the needs of students who have a latex allergy.

Allergen-Free Table

In elementary school, it is very important that an allergen-free table be available in the cafeteria. Every effort should be made to insure that the food-allergic student does not sit here alone, and that classmates with safe lunches also sit at the table. This cannot be left to chance and requires advance planning on the part of the teacher. It is equally important that the allergen-free table is not physically separated from the area of other lunch tables, and is therefore positioned in a way that does not isolate the child with food allergies. In addition, this table should be placed close to an exit door, for easy access in the event that emergency responders are called. Trash cans may be positioned away from the allergen-free table in order to reduce cross-contamination of food allergens. An EpiPen® trained staff member should be assigned to the student's lunch, and should discreetly monitor the students' activities to guard against food-sharing.

*An alternative approach by some schools is to have children who bring peanut and nut containing lunches sit at "allergen" tables. The reasoning behind this strategy is that theoretically, fewer tables in the cafeteria will be exposed to peanut/nut proteins, thus limiting the chances for skin contact reactions for students with these allergies.

Table Cleaning

There needs to be a procedure in place for thorough cleaning of all tables, including the allergen-free table. If it is the school's practice to have students clean their own lunch tables, it must be clear that the student with food allergies will only clean the allergen-free table. Secondly, a dedicated bucket and sponge must be assigned for the allergen-free table, and precautions must be made to ensure that these items are never used for the other tables. Third, a cleaning solution of water and bleach is not sufficient to remove food proteins. Soap is an integral ingredient in whatever solution will be used. A study which looked at effective products in removing peanut protein specifically found that Formula 409® , Lysol Disinfecting Wipes® , and Target® Brand Cleaner were able to effectively remove food residue from a table surface, although it was acknowledged that most commercial cleaners are sufficient in removing peanut protein.

Students with Food Allergies who Buy Lunch

If a family decides to have their child buy lunch, they should meet in advance with the Food Service Director at the school to go over food selections. The Cafeteria Director must be knowledgeable about food allergen terminology and competent to help the parent make good food choices. These meetings typically need to occur monthly to correspond with the changing lunch calendar. The U.S. Department of Agriculture (USDA) states that schools which participate in the national school lunch or breakfast programs must be in compliance with regulation 7 CFR 15b. In other words, this means that children who have documentation of special dietary needs from their physician must be able to eat food served by the school safely, even if this requires that food substitutions must be made. Clear guidelines for the Food Service Manager may be found in the USDA publication, **"Accommodating Children with Special Dietary Needs in the School Nutrition Programs."**

Some schools develop ways in which to identify students with food allergies who choose to buy lunch. For example, a system may be implemented for this purpose which includes:

1.) color-coding the lunch cards of students with food allergies, and

2.) maintaining a list of the names of these students and the foods to which they are allergic with staff at the register or check-out point. In this way, if a student has a food that should be avoided, the school employee at the check-out can observe the allergenic food before it is eaten. A safe alternative for the student can be made.

Food-allergic students who buy safe school lunches should be able to sit at the allergen-free table, along with their peers who have brought allergen-free lunches from home.

USDA Guidelines and Requirements

Food and Nutrition Service (FNS), Instruction 783-2, Revision 2, "Meal Substitutions for Medical or other Special Dietary Reasons"

The School's Responsibility:
1. The school is required to prepare safe meals of equivalent nutritional quality if requested by the family of the food-allergic student.
2. This special meal must be provided at no extra cost to the family.
3. Ingredient labels should be kept in order to reference possible food allergens, should a reaction occur.

The Family's Responsibility:
The parents need to submit documentation to the school nurse from their physician which explains:
1. The disability and why it restricts the diet.
2. The major life activity affected (*i.e.* eating).
3. The food or foods to be omitted and the foods to be used as substitutions.

Proper Storage of the Allergen-Free Table

Procedures should be implemented to ensure that the allergen-free table is not used for any other purpose once lunch is over. Schools have become quite creative in developing safe practices in this regard. Some of these include: 1.) putting a cloth over the table and placing a sign on top stating that it is "allergen-free" and should not be used, 2.) removing the table after use and placing it in a safe storage area, separate from the cafeteria, and 3.) placing duct tape on the legs of the chairs belonging to this table, so that they are not used for purposes other than lunch (the success of this initiative requires the school community to be informed of the reasons behind this practice). Avoidance procedures such as those described here will help to protect students from their allergens and will greatly reduce the likelihood of a food-induced anaphylactic event during the school day.

Adjustments to IHP Procedures for Middle and High School Students

It appears that 2.3% of teenagers have a food allergy in the United States. As food-allergic children become older and more mature, they are able to assume greater responsibilities related to the challenges presented by their health condition. Therefore, the ways in which their food allergies should be managed will differ in some ways from their younger counterparts. It is appropriate, then, to make adjustments to the student's plan for safety which allow the student greater opportunities for self-management. There is no magic age when this should automatically happen. Generally, however, most middle and high school students are ready for this type of transition. Any changes and adjustments made to a student's IHP should happen only after a careful discussion has occurred between the child and his/her parents, and an agreement is reached by all. Only then should the school nurse be approached with the intent to further discuss appropriate changes to the student's IHP. Parents and school personnel need to think of this as a journey during which time decisions and possible changes to the health plan will be made.

Although adjustments to the healthcare plan may be appropriate, it is important to remember that middle and high school students still have life-threatening food allergies at a time when, by virtue of their age, their approach to life may be changing. Teenagers often have a sense of invulnerability and consequently are more prone to risk-taking behaviors. This becomes particularly worrisome given the fact that the adolescent age is a risk factor for fatal anaphylaxis. This is also a time when many youngsters become more self-conscious, are acutely concerned with what their peers think of them, and prefer not to be treated differently in any way. This mindset can lead to reckless decision-making. A study reported in a 2003 *Pediatrics* found that of 174 adolescents surveyed who had a food allergy, only 61% always carried their EpiPen®. In order to reduce this type of attitude and risky behavior, teenagers still need to feel connected and committed to the plan for their safety. The middle and high school nurse who recognizes this will work to establish and maintain a good relationship with students who have food allergies. These students need to know that they are not alone in their efforts to avoid an allergic reaction at school, and that the health office is a place they can feel comfortable visiting if they have questions or need support.

The Epinephrine Auto-injector during Middle School and High School

First, no matter what the age, every student with a food allergy should have an EpiPen® maintained in the Health Office with the school nurse. As a student gets older, however, decisions need to be made as to whether the child with food allergies should assume the responsibility of carrying an EpiPen®, and whether he or she will self-administer epinephrine when faced with an anaphylactic event. Several factors need to be carefully considered in order to determine if the student is ready and competent to carry and/or administer this medicine. First, it is important to know if any state regulations exist which would either prohibit or allow the student to have these responsibilities. Many states do allow lifesaving medicine such as EpiPen®s and inhalers to be carried and self-administered by the student. In addition, the student's parents and allergist must be consulted regarding their advisements on this subject. Lastly, consideration should be given to the child's age, personality, maturity and desire to assume this responsibility, when making a decision of this nature. It is interesting to note that the American Academy of Pediatrics has made a recommendation that children who have experienced anaphylaxis in the past be allowed to carry their EpiPen® at all times. The EpiPen® may be kept in the pencil case of the student's notebook, or if the school allows backpacks to be carried, the student may choose to place the EpiPen® in a pocket of the student's backpack. Whichever method the student chooses, the EpiPen® must be with the student at all times, and the school nurse and the student's teachers must be aware of its location.

If a child has been given the responsibility of carrying his/her EpiPen®, it is essential that the student be given personalized instruction on its use with the physician or the school nurse. Additionally, it is important to be clear on who will administer it, should a reaction occur. If the child will self-administer, it is always advisable for a trained adult to supervise, whenever possible. It should also be clear to the student that once the EpiPen® has been self-administered, he or she must notify an adult and be transported by ambulance to a hospital. If a student takes part in after-school activities, and is a member of a team sport or perhaps a theater production, arrangements must be made for the student's EpiPen® to be easily accessed. In addition, advance planning is required to determine who will administer the EpiPen® if needed: the student, the Coach, the drama teacher, etc. These decisions and the responsibilities of everyone involved need to be clear and planned in advance. Confirmation that a cell phone, or some other form of communication is available, so that 911 may be called in the event of an emergency, is also another important safety precaution.

The Cafeteria during Middle School and High School

Although an allergen-free table is advisable for elementary school, it is unlikely that most students in middle school and high school will be interested in such a procedure. Youngsters at this age generally prefer to sit where they want. That being said, students should still practice good hand washing to avoid allergen exposure, their EpiPen® must be readily available, and they should not eat any food unless it was prepared at home or they are physically able to read an ingredient list. Lastly, it is still recommended that an EpiPen® trained staff member be present in a middle school and high school cafeteria.

TRANSITION FROM ELEMENTARY SCHOOL TO THE MIDDLE SCHOOL

A student's transition from a nurturing elementary school environment to a middle school setting presents quite a challenge. This is an age when the student is trying desperately to gain independence. They begin pushing away from parents and teachers who have been watching over them and are now attempting to gain acceptance from their peers. The challenge with this age group is to provide a safe environment while teaching and encouraging the student to self-manage his/her allergies. Working to accomplish this task, I keep in mind the guidelines set by Dr. Hugh Sampson MD (Allergist/Immunologist) - Awareness - Avoidance - Education - Preparedness.

Awareness is accomplished by informing staff members, fellow classmates, bus drivers, coaches, etc. about the student's food allergies and what they need to do to reduce risk of exposure. This is done at the beginning of the school year before the student arrives in the building.

Avoidance is handled greatly by the student. The staff is notified not to reward students with food and to avoid the use of food for school projects. If food is to be used for any reason, it must be cleared by the school nurse or the student's parents, well in advance. Cafeteria food is screened by trained employees. Labels are diligently read and any foods that are unsafe are eliminated from the menu and snack bar.

Education is multifaceted. Everyone involved with the student needs to be educated regarding food allergies. An "Individual Healthcare Plan" is developed in collaboration with the parents, school nurse and guidance counselor and then shared with the staff. I like to use this time to educate the student, as well. The student needs to be reminded not to share food and NEVER eat anything without reading the ingredient label. If the student is involved in the label-reading process, it will encourage growth and independence to prepare him for the future. In the event an EpiPen® needs to be used at school, I like to utilize this opportunity to teach the student to self-inject. This gives the student a great sense of empowerment knowing they are able to accomplish this task.

Preparedness involves having an "Emergency Action Plan" in place, practicing the plan, storing medication in an easily accessible place, and sharing this information with all staff that interacts with the student, as well as teaching everyone how to use an EpiPen®.

It is important to look at each student individually, assess their needs, set policies to insure risk reduction and create a safe environment for the student at school.

Terri McDonough, BSN, RN, Middle School Nurse, Hingham, Massachusetts

STEP TWO: EDUCATION

It is imperative for a school community to understand the nature of food allergies and anaphylaxis, in order for the individuals within that community to understand and become proponents of food allergy management protocols and procedures in place. Education, therefore, becomes a necessary and important second step in our 3-Step Management Plan. The National Association of School Nurses (NASN), in their study, "Impact of Food Allergies on School Nursing Practices", which was presented in the October, 2004 *Journal of School Nursing,* concluded that training of school staff on food allergies is critical as a preventive measure to appropriately manage the potential for anaphylaxis at school. Therefore, in order for teachers and school staff to recognize the symptoms of a food-allergic reaction, become familiar with the ways in which an individual may become exposed to their allergens, and become competent in planning preventive measures, **comprehensive training** on this subject must be provided.

General Education for Food Allergies and Anaphylaxis

The content of a thorough training program should include general information on the nature of food allergies and anaphylaxis. Specifically, attendees should come away from the training with a basic understanding of the definition of a true food allergy, and how it differs from a food intolerance. They should understand the symptoms of a food allergy reaction, including the body systems that may be involved, such as the skin, the gastrointestinal, respiratory and cardiovascular systems. School staff should also be familiar with the signs and symptoms of anaphylaxis, including the concept of how quickly a food-allergic reaction may escalate into anaphylaxis. The ways in which a person may become exposed to allergen(s), especially within the context of the school environment, should be covered, such as through ingestion, skin contact, inhalation and cross-contamination (refer to information covered in Chapter One).

A **general training** program on food allergies should also cover the protocols currently being employed by the school to manage food allergies, so that school personnel are fully aware of procedures in place and their role and responsibilities as they relate to those procedures. This would be the time to indicate where EpiPen®s are stored (never in a locked cabinet during school hours), and who, on staff, has been trained to administer one, should the need arise. A review of preventive procedures being implemented throughout the school environment should be presented, such as in the cafeteria, on the playground and at recess, on the bus and on field trips, and during before and after school-sponsored events. Information needs to be shared during this general training program regarding written school and/or district policy on managing life-threatening allergies, including information on how such documents may be referenced. This would also be the time to review disability laws, such as Section

504 of The Rehabilitation Act of 1973 and The Americans with
Disabilities Act of 1990, which protect the rights of individuals with
life-threatening food allergies (see Chapter 4 for more information
on this).

This general training is best planned and presented by the school
nurse. In situations where there is not a school nurse, the training
may be provided by a school-affiliated physician. Help in planning
the content of this type of education can usually be provided for
by personnel within the State Department of Public Health. Ideally,
all staff members should be present for this training, including
teachers, school administrators, specialist teachers, auxiliary staff,
cafeteria and bus personnel. As discussed earlier in this chapter,
the high percentage of individuals not previously known to have
an allergic condition and who have experienced anaphylaxis while
at school, means that all staff should be educated to recognize the
signs of an allergic reaction. This type of education will also give
school administration and staff the knowledge they need to plan and
implement comprehensive food allergy management procedures.

It is also strongly recommended that the parent and student
communities receive education on food allergies and how they
impact the school environment, as well. A Parent-Teacher
Organization (PTO) meeting and a classroom activity designed for
this purpose, respectively, provide excellent opportunities for this
type of education. Once parents have a better understanding of how
easily a student can be exposed to their allergens, and how severe
an allergic reaction may become, they are typically more supportive
of endeavors to keep these students safe. Furthermore, when this
subject is handled with sensitivity and in an age-appropriate manner,
most children seem to respond by becoming quite protective of their
food-allergic classmates.

When all members of a school community acquire a basic knowledge
and understanding of the complexities of this health issue, it tends to
enhance their acceptance and cooperation with regards to reasonable
requests made by the school in its efforts to manage food allergies.
This, in turn, will not only help to minimize a student's risk of

experiencing a food-induced allergic reaction, or worse, anaphylaxis, but it will also allow the student with this special healthcare need to benefit fully from all aspects of his/her school program. Once again, timing is important. Ideally, training and education should take place at the start of the school year.

SAMPLE STAFF SCHOOL FOOD ALLERGY MANAGEMENT TRAINING OUTLINE

I. FOOD ALLERGY OVERVIEW

    A. Current U.S. Food Allergy Statistics
    B. Definition of a True Food Allergy vs. a Food Sensitivity
    C. Symptoms of an Allergic Reaction
    D. Anaphylaxis as Defined by the National Institute of Health
    E. The "Big Eight" Food Allergens
    F. Routes of Exposure

II. GUIDELINES FOR SCHOOL FOOD ALLERGY MANAGEMENT

    A. Step One—Avoidance
        1.) Individual Healthcare Plan
        2.) 504 Plans

    B. Step Two—Education
        1.) Protocols/Procedures in Place
        2.) District Policy
        3.) Overview of Disability Laws

    C. Step Three—Response
        1.) Epinephrine by Auto-Injector (EpiPen®) Administration Training
        2.) Emergency Treatment Plan

III. SUMMARY OF GOALS AND STAFF RESPONSIBILITIES

IMPORTANCE OF EDUCATION

I am the nurse leader in a school district with an ever increasing number of students with life threatening allergies. When the parent of a child with allergies sends them off to school for the first time, the experience can be overwhelming and frightening. In addition, it is extremely important for parents of non-allergic children to understand the impact a life threatening allergy can have on everyday activities. Education has proven to be the most powerful and effective tool that we can have in our school community. Education of parents, students and staff has helped to provide not only understanding of the law and rights of students but, more importantly, it has provided an increased community-wide diligence in ensuring that necessary accommodations for the food allergic student are respected.

Gail Kelley RN, Nurse Leader,
Dedham Public Schools, Massachusetts

STEP THREE—RESPONSE

"A community is like a ship; everyone ought to be prepared to take the helm." Henrik Ibsen

---

EFFECTIVE FOOD ALLERGY MANAGEMENT REQUIRES TWO DISTINCT HEALTHCARE PLANS:

1.) A Plan for Prevention (Individualized Healthcare Plan)
2.) A Plan for Treatment of an Allergic Reaction (Emergency Treatment Plan)

Epinephrine Auto-injector Training

There remains the unfortunate possibility that a student with food allergies may, at some point during his/her career as a student, experience some type of an allergic reaction while at school. Despite educational initiatives and the existence of well-intentioned procedures to prevent exposure to allergens, we are all human, and, despite the best of intentions, errors can be made. Consequently, a competent response plan is a necessary component of any food allergy management plan. This requires that a school have protocols and procedures in place to ensure that:

1.) Staff receive adequate training in the proper administration of the epinephrine auto-injector (EpiPen®).

2.) The EpiPen® is readily accessible.

3.) Each student with a food allergy has a written Emergency Treatment Plan

4.) There is thorough documentation of each event when epinephrine by auto-injector has been administered.

The school nurse is the individual at school with the most medical training, and therefore, should be the primary person responsible for administering epinephrine to a student experiencing anaphylaxis. The school nurse, however, may only work part time, or for other reasons, may not be readily available when a medical emergency presents itself. Because of this possibility, it is critical that additional staff members at a school accept the responsibility of treating a student who is experiencing anaphylaxis, and also agree to be trained in the proper administration of epinephrine by auto-injector. How many individuals should receive this training? The simple and most direct answer to this question is that *all* staff members within a school community should be encouraged to receive EpiPen® training. Given the fact that a significant number of school-aged children have a food allergy, it makes good sense that all adult school personnel be prepared to respond to a student experiencing anaphylaxis, if they were to ever encounter this type of medical emergency. Unfortunately, while most school employees do not hesitate to receive CPR training, not everyone feels as comfortable with the idea of administering an EpiPen®. If epinephrine were made in pill form, chances are that most people would not hesitate to respond and give it to the person in need. To alleviate the fear and concern which some school staff may have, the following information is suggested as "food for thought":

- It is important to understand that the EpiPen® was designed by Dey Laboratories so that it would be simple and easy to use, regardless of whether a person has any medical training,

- The school nurse may not always be present and/or available with the sufficient time needed to respond to someone having anaphylaxis,

- Epinephrine will not cause any serious side effects in an otherwise healthy person,

- If liability is a concern, it should be understood that most states have Good Samaritan laws. This means that if a staff member, in good faith, administered the EpiPen® to an individual experiencing anaphylaxis, and in so doing, did what he or she believed could be done to help the person in the throes of a medical emergency, based on the intent of the Good Samaritan law, this staff member should be protected from civil liability issues. If this is an issue of concern, it is advisable to check the laws and their wording in your state.

- Epinephrine is the only treatment which will reverse the symptoms of anaphylaxis, and therefore, administering it promptly could truly save someone's life (see Chapter 1).

State Regulations for EpiPen® Administration

In most states, the Department of Health has **regulations** to provide standards for maintaining safety in the administration of epinephrine by auto-injector. When a state has regulations which provide for an unlicensed school staff member to administer epinephrine by auto-injector in an emergency, the school nurse is typically required to conduct EpiPen® training for this individual. The term "unlicensed" may be defined here as anyone without a nursing license. For example, in Massachusetts, all public and private schools that intend to permit this responsibility to unlicensed personnel must fill out an application to register with the Massachusetts Department of Public Health for this purpose. A condition included within MA regulation 105 CMR 210 is the requirement that, in addition to training these individuals in the correct technique to administer the EpiPen®, the school must also have " . . . a plan for comprehensive risk reduction for the student, including preventing exposure to specific allergens." The presence of this requirement signals the Department's commitment to the immense importance preventive measures play in a school's efforts to manage its students' food allergies.

Some State Departments of Health also provide a curriculum for their school nurses to use as a means to facilitate this training. In Massachusetts, the Department of Public Health has developed a curriculum for this purpose, and has also included an "Epinephrine Competency Checklist" to be completed by trainees at the end of their training. Successful completion of the "Checklist" serves a dual purpose: school nurses can feel confident that the proper technique to administer the EpiPen® has been learned, and recently trained staff members can have the confidence that they are sufficiently prepared to respond to this medical emergency, should the need arise.

Recommended Guidelines for EpiPen® Administration

The following are **guidelines** which should be considered for inclusion in EpiPen® training conducted for unlicensed school personnel:

- It is strongly recommended for each student who has a food allergy, that an adult staff member is assigned the responsibility of being the "first responder" to administer the EpiPen® to that student, should he or she experience an anaphylactic reaction. In addition to this "first responder", who is usually the school nurse, there should be a second EpiPen® trained staff member, usually the classroom teacher, assigned to each food-allergic student. This concept of a "chain of command" of first responders helps to ensure that in the event that a student has anaphylaxis, and the first responder (school nurse) is not available, a second Epi-trained individual (classroom teacher) understands that it is his/her role to administer the EpiPen®. Many schools find that a chain of command which is three-deep works best.

- For any staff member who will have the responsibility of administering the EpiPen® to a student, should the need arise, it is helpful to arrange a meeting between that staff member and the student to begin to develop face recognition and a comfortable relationship between the two parties. This activity can contribute greatly to a shy or reticent child's willingness to seek help from an adult whom they have previously met.

- School staff should understand that once they determine that a person is experiencing the symptoms of anaphylaxis, it is critical that the EpiPen® be administered right away. A study which looked at the effectiveness of epinephrine in relieving the symptoms of anaphylaxis found that when the EpiPen® was given within 30 minutes of the onset of the first symptom, symptoms resolved promptly. Furthermore, the American Academy of Pediatrics reported in their Position Paper dated March, 2007, that a delay in giving epinephrine was associated with fatal anaphylaxis. It should be understood that epinephrine can not be given too early, but it can be given too late.

- The effects of epinephrine last anywhere from ten to twenty minutes, and there may be times when a second dose may be required if the person's symptoms persist or worsen. The American Academy of Pediatrics recommends that a second dose of epinephrine may be given as early as five to twenty minutes if the first dose was not effective in reversing symptoms, or if the symptoms continue to worsen.

- Once the EpiPen® has been administered, protocols should be in place for a staff member to immediately call 911 so that an emergency response team may be sent to transport the individual to the hospital. When calling 911, it is very important to identify that the person is having anaphylaxis so that the EMTs can be triaged appropriately. Be aware in advance as to whether or not the EMTs carry epinephrine—not all states allow this. In locations where this is not allowed, it becomes critical to send a second EpiPen® in the ambulance with an EpiPen® trained school staff member. It is recommended that once treated, the individual remain in the hospital setting for four hours, as a safeguard in case a biphasic reaction occurs.

- A thorough report must be written by the school nurse to document all pertinent information related to this emergency event. This report should be kept on file at school and in addition, should also be submitted to the State Department of Health, if such a procedure is in place.

- EpiPen®s should be checked periodically to insure that the expiration date for the medicine has not passed. This responsibility is usually carried out by the school nurse. The medicine should also be examined to make sure that it has not become discolored, which can happen as a result of its exposure to extreme cold or hot temperatures. The color of the epinephrine can be seen through the side of the auto-injector device, and it should appear clear. Transporting EpiPen®s in an insulated bag, such as an insulated lunch container, is an easy and practical way to help protect the medicine from temperature extremes.

Accessibility of Epinephrine

It would seem logical to expect that lifesaving medicine, such as the EpiPen®, would be kept in close proximity to someone who has a history of food allergies and anaphylaxis. It appears, however, that in practice, this is not always the case. The study entitled, "Impact of Food Allergies on School Nursing Practice", which was referenced earlier in this chapter, also reported that 90% of the school nurses interviewed kept their EpiPens® primarily in their office, and not in other areas of the school environment, such as in the classroom or cafeteria. The study concluded that school staff was not adequately prepared to effectively manage food allergies at school, that epinephrine needs to be stored in safe locations that allow for timely access for its administration, and that it never should be kept in a locked cabinet. It also made note that schools have been held legally responsible for failing to recognize and treat an allergic reaction promptly.

Optimally, two epinephrine auto-injectors should be prescribed and available at school for every student diagnosed with a food allergy. Realistically, providing a school with two devices may be financially difficult for some families. Whenever possible, however, it is advisable for each student to have two epinephrine auto-injectors on hand in the event that a biphasic reaction occurs, or in the event that the first auto-injector malfunctions for some reason. In addition, there also should be a standing order of both doses of epinephrine (0.15 mg. and 0.3 mg.) for the nurse to use in the event that an individual with undiagnosed food allergies experiences anaphylaxis.

A school should be prepared to store epinephrine in safe locations which would also allow for the prompt treatment of an allergic reaction. This means that *a student's EpiPen® should be kept where the student is at most risk for anaphylaxis, AND where it can be accessed within a matter of minutes.* The EpiPen® and related medicines should be kept in the school nurse's office, and never under lock and key during school hours. It is also recommended that another EpiPen® be kept in the student's classroom. Many schools and families choose to have a third EpiPen® stored safely in the cafeteria.

In addition to the EpiPen® stored in the Health Room, The American Academy of Asthma, Allergy & Immunology states in their 1998 Position Paper, "Anaphylaxis in Schools and Other Childcare Settings", that "For younger children, the epinephrine device should be kept in the classroom and passed from teacher to teacher as the child moves through the school (e.g., from classroom to music to PE to lunch)." This strategy may cause concern for some school officials who believe that with this scenario, the possibility exists for the teacher to forget to transport the EpiPen®, thus putting the child at risk if an allergic reaction were to occur. It is important to point out, however, that schools that have opted to use this strategy have found the pros far outweigh the cons, and that this method, in fact, works extremely well. School nurses with whom I have spoken who choose to utilize this strategy, and have the EpiPen® passed between school staff members, are consistently enthusiastic about how well this system actually works. Once this procedure has been established, it becomes a matter of routine. On the rare occasion that the medicine has been forgotten, it has been reported that in almost every case, inevitably, one of the students in the class would signal its absence before the classroom was exited!

We know that students travel beyond the confines of the school building when they go out for recess, when they play a sport at another school, and when the enrichment curriculum includes a field trip offsite. Consequently, thought and planning must also be spent determining the location and manner in which epinephrine will be transported in these circumstances, and who will be responsible for administering the medicine, if required. Ultimately, a student's EpiPen® must be equally accessible regardless of whether the student is inside or outside of the school environment.

The Emergency Treatment Plan

When a student experiences anaphylaxis, it is extremely beneficial for the first responder to have a clear sense of the best way to go about treating the student. Every student who has a diagnosed food allergy must have an individualized, written Emergency Treatment Plan (ETP) for the medical treatment of an allergic reaction at school (this plan has also been called an Emergency Action Plan, a Food Allergy Action Plan, an Allergy Action Plan, etc.). No matter its name, the student's emergency treatment plan should outline, in a clear, step-by-step format, the specific treatment plan to follow. The ETP should also include the following:

- Identifying information for the student (name, date of birth, address, grade)

- Relevant medical history (Asthma, eczema, foods to which the student is allergic, symptoms of an allergic reaction previously presented)

- A current, color photo of the student

- The physician's signature, with the date

- The parent's signature, with the date

- Emergency contact information (parent's home and cell phone numbers, physician's office phone number)

The physician's signature signifies that this plan of treatment has been endorsed by the physician. The ETP should be reviewed and signed by the school nurse and the parents prior to the start of the school year and it should be reviewed and updated annually. Whenever a student is treated with epinephrine, 911 must be called and the student should be transported to the hospital emergency department. The student's parents should also be called and informed of the name and location of the medical facility where their child has been taken.

Copies of the ETP should be kept wherever the EpiPen® is kept, such as in the nurse's office, with the medicine in the classroom, or with the medicine in the cafeteria, for example. Laminating the ETP is strongly recommended because it will help to preserve it over the course of the year. These plans should not be posted for the general public to see. Therefore, care must be taken to place copies of the ETP in locations where only staff who have a reasonable "need to know" may view them. In other words, in order to protect the student and family's right to privacy, the ETP should not be posted in open places where other students and parents are able to read it. (For more information on this, refer to Chapter 4, "The Laws".) Examples of three sample Emergency Treatment Plan forms are included in the Supplement section at the end of this chapter.

KEYS TO ENHANCE EFFECTIVE MANAGEMENT

It is important to understand that there are ways in which to dramatically enhance the success of school food allergy management efforts, while also allowing for the process to be less stressful or adversarial for everyone. Programs which appear to achieve the greatest productivity are those which appreciate the importance of the following:

1.) Adopt a **proactive** approach and make plans in advance, whenever possible.

It is extremely important to be proactive and whenever possible, plan ahead. The goal is to have everything in place by the first day of school. Therefore, parents and school staff need to allow for a reasonable amount of time to discuss all aspects of the child's food allergy management plan. This is not the time to be last minute. Scheduling a meeting may take time. In addition, school staff need to dedicate a fair amount of time for these planning meetings. By planning ahead, and allowing sufficient time for discussion, there will be less likelihood that critical considerations for the safety of the food-allergic child will be overlooked.

2.) Develop the attitude that this must be truly viewed as a **partnership** between all parties.

It is critical that the family and school establish a healthy partnership. The need for a successful collaboration is simple: school personnel know their environment best and parents know their child best. When working as a unit rather than as separate parts, all bases will more likely be covered. There may be times, and for a variety of reasons, when this may become difficult. It is important for both parties to stay focused and keep in mind that what is most important is the health and safety of a child. A working relationship that is team-based will greatly facilitate the development of effective strategies for food allergy management at school.

3.) Maintain regular and open **communication** between everyone who is involved in efforts to keep the food-allergic child safe.

Clear and open communication is the third factor which is paramount to success. The simple truth is that we can't know what we haven't been told. Both parents and school staff must feel comfortable asking questions of one another. Similarly, it is important for each party to be an active and careful listener so that information shared is heard and understood. This format allows for an important exchange of ideas and also an opportunity for clarification, when needed. When something is unclear, ask for further explanation. Lack of communication or misunderstood communication could cause confusion and potentially errors that have serious consequences.

It is also extremely important to remember to include the student with food allergies in discussions which pertain to the student's safety. Parents, teachers, nurses, etc., may, at times, become so immersed in their planning, that they forget to inform the child/student what procedures will be followed. Students with food allergies need to be "in-the-know" in an age-appropriate way. They need to have confidence that there is a plan for their safety at school, they need to understand who to approach when they have questions, and they need to be familiar with what their role will be within the plan or strategy.

Lastly, utilize all of the many ways in which we may communicate with one another, whether it is through in-person conversations or meetings, utilizing email or the traditional mail system, or the telephone—whatever it takes! The venue is not important; what *is* important is that an atmosphere is established that allows for questions to be asked, and answers heard.

4.) Pay attention to **"high risk"** times, to ensure that safe protocols are being practiced.

A high risk time may be defined as any activity or procedure which interrupts or is different from the regular, daily routine, because this is usually when important safety details can be overlooked. Examples of this would be holidays, field trips, substitute teachers, special school events, fire drills, etc.

5.) Make sure to conduct an **evaluation** of the procedures within the student's IHP.

A regular evaluation of a student's IHP is an important way to ensure that the procedures being followed are appropriate, clear and effective in their intent to enhance the student's safety while he or she is engaged in school activities and programs. An evaluation should take place whenever the student experiences an allergic reaction at school, in order to determine what changes need to be made to avoid a future reaction. Additionally, the content of the IHP should be reviewed at the end of each school year so that adjustments may be made, when appropriate, which reflect changes in the student's growth and development. A thorough review of the plan will also help determine if the accommodations within the plan have been reasonable and effective.

Conclusion

An effective school food allergy management program requires careful planning. Parents and schools must adopt a collaborative and proactive approach in their efforts to manage food allergies at school. By working together in a concerted effort, it is possible to develop and implement reasonable accommodations meant to keep food-allergic children safe at school *and* to successfully handle an anaphylactic reaction in case one should occur. In this way, an atmosphere will be promoted which will allow the student the opportunity to experience all aspects of his/her education. With the appropriate knowledge and planning, the goals of food allergy management at school can be achieved.

Too many children are having allergic reactions and anaphylaxis while at school in the United States. Each reaction is traumatic for the student who experiences it, for those who witness it, and for the people who treat the child in the throes of this real, life threatening event. Apathy, denial or indifference should not be an option. The strategies included in this chapter will help keep children with food allergies safe at school because they are effective, reasonable and easily implemented.

"Always bear in mind that your own resolution to success is more important than any other thing."

Abraham Lincoln

►**ADDITIONAL RESOURCES USEFUL FOR SCHOOL FOOD ALLERGY MANAGEMENT:**

- **The School Food Allergy Program**, a binder for educators developed by *The Food Allergy and Anaphylaxis Network* (FAAN). www.foodallergy.org.

- **How to C.A.R.E.™ For Students with Food Allergies: What Educators Should Know**, a free, online program developed by FAI, FAAN, and Anaphylaxis Canada. www. allergyready.com.

- **NASN** online food allergy toolkit for school nurses developed by the National Association of School Nurses, Food Allergy and Anaphylaxis Network, and the National School Board Association, with a grant from the Centers for Disease Control. www.nasn.org/ToolsResources/ FoodAllergyandAnaphylaxis.

SUPPLEMENTAL MATERIALS

RECOMMENDED STANDARDS FOR SCHOOL FOOD ALLERGY MANAGEMENT

FOCUS AREA: THE PARENTS

Parents are the "Information Givers" and primary educators of their child. They need to:

- Notify the school of their child's food allergies before the start of the school year.

- Provide up-to-date medical documentation from the child's physician, including physician's orders and all paperwork requested by the school.

- Supply all medications necessary, including an insulated bag and/or backpack to carry the medicines from one location to another.

- Provide information about their child's food allergy, including signs and symptoms of previous allergic reactions, and related medical history.

- Work with the school nurse collaboratively to develop the best procedures for use in their child's Individual Healthcare Plan (IHP).

- Provide their child's physician-approved Emergency Treatment Plan.

- Provide contact information in the event of an emergency or question.

- Meet with the teacher to discuss their child's IHP, and safe procedures regarding food used for snacks, celebrations and in the curriculum.

- Coordinate safe foods with the teacher and Room Parent.

- Keep a supply of safe foods at school, at all times.

- Assist in Peer/Parent education.

- Be available as a resource.

- Attend all field trips, whenever possible.

- Educate their child in understanding the foods to which the child is allergic, food allergen terminology, and what the child's responsibilities will be within the IHP.

- Meet with the school nurse in spring in order to evaluate appropriate procedures to be included in the IHP for the next school year.

FOCUS AREA: THE STUDENT

The student needs to practice age-appropriate responsibilities, including:

- No food sharing, ever. The only exception to this would be when and if the student is able to read an ingredient list and can make an informed decision. For youngsters, their mantra needs to be "If I can't read it, I won't eat it!"

- Eat only approved foods/drinks, according to the IHP.

- Notify an adult right away when an allergic reaction is suspected.

- Understand how an EpiPen® works, and his/her role in administering it.

*(For young children, it is recommended that the school nurse or a trained adult administer the EpiPen®; for older children who have been given permission to self-administer, it is important that the school nurse or a trained adult supervise.)

- Understand where the EpiPen®(s) will be kept, and what role, if any, the student will have if the medication will be transported.

For elementary school, it is recommended that trained staff carry the EpiPen®; for middle school and high school, it is recommended that the student carry the EpiPen® either in a pencil case located in a notebook which must be carried all the time, or in a zippered section of the student's backpack, which must be carried all the time. It is essential that the school nurse and EpiPen® trained school personnel be advised of the EpiPen® location when it is carried by the student. For older students attending school-sponsored events before/after school, it is recommended that the student carry the epinephrine auto-injector.

- Follow good hand washing practices (recommended whenever the classroom is entered and before eating).

- Understand allergen terminology (age appropriate).

- Wear a Medic Alert bracelet.

FOCUS AREA: THE SCHOOL NURSE

The School Nurse is the initiator and implementer of the student's Individual Healthcare Plan. In addition, the school nurse is the point of contact for all school personnel involved in the student's safety procedures, and must be proactive in all efforts. This will require that the school nurse:

- Be familiar with all state regulations regarding EpiPen® administration delegation and state guidelines regarding food allergy management.

- Follow up on submitted medical documentation of a student's food allergy, with the student's parents.

- Work to develop a strong partnership with the parents and the student.

- Work with the student's parents to develop the IHP before the start of the school year.

- Adopt a multi-disciplinary approach and arrange a Team Meeting with all school personnel who will have direct contact with the student in order to review the IHP and ETP and to discuss the staff's role and responsibilities within the student's IHP and ETP, before or at the start of the school year.

- Oversee the implementation of all aspects of the student's IHP.

- Conduct an In-Service training prior to the start of the school year, to *all* school staff regarding:

  1. General education on food allergies

  2. Symptoms and treatment of an allergic/anaphylactic reaction

  3. School procedures intended to reduce/avoid contact with food allergens

  4. Emergency response protocols

- Conduct EpiPen® administration training to all school staff who will have *direct contact with the studen*t, in accordance with State regulations.

- Maintain the EpiPen® and any related medicine, in an accessible location in the Health Room, and never in a locked cabinet during the school day. Keep the Emergency Treatment Plan wherever the EpiPen® is stored.

- Maintain a copy of the Individual Healthcare Plan in the Health Room.

- Check the expiration dates of the EpiPen® auto-injector.

- Educate new personnel as necessary.

- Check-in with a substitute teacher assigned to the student's class, whenever possible.

- Make available written protocols regarding the student's IHP/ETP for a substitute nurse to follow whenever the school nurse is absent.

- Evaluate the procedures within the IHP whenever a reaction occurs and in the spring to plan for the subsequent year.

- Following treatment of anaphylaxis with epinephrine, file a report with the state Department of Public Health (or appropriate agency). Hold a follow-up meeting with the family and school staff to review the incident and possible adjustments to the IHP and ETP to prevent future incidents.

FOCUS AREA: SCHOOL ADMINISTRATION (Principal)

The school principal sets the tone for a positive environment by demonstrating a commitment to school food allergy management procedures and protocols and will:

- Work to insure there is a full time nurse.

- Assign the student to a teacher who is willing to be EpiPen® trained, who is willing to administer the EpiPen® should the student experience anaphylaxis, and who is willing to follow the student's IHP procedures.

- Coordinate a meeting between the parents and the student's teacher prior to the start of the school year.

- Send a letter to all classroom parents informing them that a student with life threatening food allergies will be in their child's class.

- Writes letters as needed to inform the school community (parents and school personnel) of food allergy protocols in place.

- Work with the school nurse and the parents of the food-allergic student to insure that all school-sponsored events, including those planned before and after school, will allow for the safe participation of the student.

- Include information on school food allergen guidelines in the School Handbook.

- Put procedures into place to address allergen-free procedures when outside organizations use school space for meetings/ events.

- Provide for school-wide emergency response protocols to include anaphylaxis.

- Implement a "Zero Tolerance" Policy regarding all threats/ harassment. Address all incidents of bullying promptly and decisively.

- Understand and follow federal and state laws that apply to this issue.

FOCUS AREA: TEACHER / THE CLASSROOM

The goal of the classroom teacher is to keep the child with food allergies safe within the learning environment. The classroom teacher plays a critical role in the student's daily food allergy management and will:

- Receive general food allergy education and be trained in EpiPen® administration and be willing to administer the EpiPen®, when required.

- Participate in a meeting with the school nurse and parent prior to/at the beginning of the school year to review student's IHP and ETP. Understand his/her role and responsibilities in each healthcare plan.

- Maintain the student's EpiPen® and ETP in a safe location in the classroom, if requested.

- Understand the teacher's responsibility regarding the transportation of the EpiPen®.

- Establish an allergen-free classroom, if required. Review, in advance, any projects in curriculum involving food, make safe substitutions when necessary.

- Establish safe procedures for snack, birthday, holidays.

- Oversee hand washing procedures, as stated in the student's IHP.

- Clean desk/table surfaces, as necessary, per student's IHP.

- Use non-food items for rewards.

- Use a communication device for contact with the Health Room both in and outside of the school building (e.g. intercom, cell phone, walkie-talkie.).

- Transport the medical bag which contains the EpiPen® and ETP outside for recess on the playground.

- Plan for the student's assignment to an allergen-free table in the cafeteria, if requested. Make arrangements to insure the student will not sit alone.

- Plan for the student's safety for field trips, including notification to the student's parents, in advance of the trip (Refer to "Field Trip Focus Area" for more specific information).

- Place the student's IHP and ETP in a folder where it will be clearly visible for a Substitute Teacher.

- Plan for Parent and Peer education.

- Place an "Allergen-Free" sign outside classroom, if specified in student's IHP.

- During a fire drill, carry the student's EpiPen® and related medicine.

- Send reminder notices at holiday times.

- Address harassment related to food allergies immediately.

FOCUS AREA: SUBSTITUTE TEACHERS

When a substitute teacher is in charge of the classroom, this may be considered a "high risk" time, and procedures must be in place which facilitates the safety of the student with food allergies.

- The substitute teacher will read information posted in the **"Substitute Teacher Folder"** which will include the student's IHP and information on the location of the student's EpiPen® and ETP. Color-coding this notebook may make it easier to locate.

- In elementary school it is recommended that office staff arranging for a substitute teacher for a class with a food-allergic student will notify the school nurse at the start of the day.

- The nurse should check with the substitute teacher to answer any questions regarding food allergy procedures.

FOCUS AREA: SPECIALISTS

Specialist teachers include such areas as music, art, computer, library, etc. These school personnel will have direct contact with the students who have food allergy during the school day, and are therefore responsible for their safety and wellbeing. They should:

- Attend general food allergy education sessions, be made aware of food allergy protocols at school, and attend anaphylaxis training.

- Understand their role as stated in the student's IHP, and responsibilities related to the student's EpiPen®.

- For Computer Class, the computer keyboard should be wiped down prior to the food-allergic student's use, if stated in the student's IHP.

- In Art and Music, precautions should be made to insure that no projects include the student's allergens.

FOCUS AREA: FIELD TRIPS

Field trips, because they present an interruption to the normal, daily school routine, are considered "high risk" times. Thoughtful planning is required to ensure that a field trip will not involve food allergens that will pose a risk to the safety of the student with food allergies. The teacher planning the trip will:

- Notify the school nurse as soon as a field trip is planned so that arrangements for the student's medicines may be made.

- Invite the parent of the food-allergic child, in a timely manner, to attend all field trips (for elementary school).

- Make sure that a nurse or an EpiPen® trained adult staff member will be present on the field trip.

- Make sure the EpiPen® and the ETP will be carried by the EpiPen® trained staff member, or by the student, if appropriate.

- Have a communication device, such as a cell phone, available on the trip in the event a medical emergency occurs.

- Determine, with the school nurse, the name and phone number of the closest hospital prior to the field trip.

- If lunch or snacks are to be eaten while on the field trip, consider requesting that no food allergens are sent, especially peanut/nut products, and "powdery" cheese foods, if students on the trip have peanut, nut or milk allergies.

- Make sure wet wipes are available to be used after food has been eaten.

- Enforce a strict "No Eating" policy on the bus.

FOCUS AREA: GYM

Gym class represents a less controlled environment as compared with other areas within the school, and that implicitly denotes an increased risk to the safety of the food allergic student. Specifically, activities in gym usually include interactions between students that are physical, and there is a significant amount of equipment that is typically shared amongst the entire student population. Both of these factors can contribute to exposure to food allergens through skin contact and cross-contamination. Proactive procedures must be implemented to reduce these risks, including:

- The gym teacher will receive general food allergy education and should be trained in EpiPen® administration.

- The EpiPen® and ETP will be available at all times, including when class is held outside.

- A form of communication, such as an intercom, cell phone or walkie-talkie will be available, including when gym is held outside.

- The gym teacher will follow any other procedures as stated in the student's IHP.

FOCUS AREA: THE CAFETERIA

The cafeteria presents an area of the school where a substantial amount of food is present every day. Because of this, precautions must be taken to protect the student with food allergies from coming into contact with their food allergens. The Food Service Director must:

- Be familiar with the laws that pertain to students with life threatening food allergies, and be in compliance with their requirements (USDA Federal Regulation 7 CFR 15b).

- Work with families who would like their child to buy lunch, and help them to make safe choices. Safe food substitutions, at no extra cost to the family should be provided, and food product labels should be kept for a reasonable amount of time, as a reference, should an allergic reaction occur.

- Develop a system to identify students with life-threatening food allergies who buy lunch, while also maintaining their privacy (see Chapter 4 for information on FERPA requirements).

- Provide general food allergy education for all cafeteria staff. Cafeteria staff should be knowledgeable about the "Big Eight" food allergens, and signs and symptoms of an allergic reaction.

- Provide staff education on proper food handling to avoid cross-contamination of food being prepared or served. Cafeteria staff must understand the ways in which food allergens can come into contact with one another, and how cross-contamination of food allergens can cause severe allergic reactions and anaphylaxis for students with food allergies.

- Provide guidance and supervision regarding proper cleaning procedures for all pots, pans, kitchen utensils and counter surfaces.

- Cooperate with other school personnel regarding procedures for the use and storage of allergen-free tables.

- Consider reducing or eliminating the sale of peanut and nut products in the cafeteria.

- Maintain a file of ingredient lists of processed and prepared foods from vendors.

FOCUS AREA: MAINTENANCE

Maintenance staff has the unique ability to insure that surfaces are clean and void of offending food allergens, and to help with other procedures meant to reduce a food-allergic student's risk of experiencing an allergic reaction at school. This can be accomplished when maintenance staff:

- Receive general food allergy education.

- Read ingredient labels of cleaning products, including soaps used, to insure that they do not contain food allergens (e.g., nut oils, milk products, etc.).

- Store the allergen-free table in the cafeteria as stated in student's IHP.

- Carry out responsibilities for thorough cleaning of all areas in the school, understanding that a solution of bleach and water is insufficient at removing food allergen proteins.

FOCUS AREA: BUS TRANSPORTATION

School personnel are responsible for the safety of their students starting at the beginning of the school day until the end of the day. For many students, the start of their day begins with the bus ride into school. Safety precautions must be taken for all students who ride on the bus, including those with food allergies. This can be difficult when a bus company is hired by the school, however the fact remains that the school has a responsibility and obligation to make arrangements which meet the needs of these students. This can be accomplished when The Supervisor of Bus Transportation makes:

- Arrangements for the bus drivers to receive general food allergy education and training in EpiPen® administration.

Training is usually conducted by the school district's Head Nurse or Nurse Supervisor.

- Arrangements for students with food allergies to be driven by bus drivers who have received EpiPen® training, whenever possible.

- Arrangements for the student's Emergency Treatment Plan (ETP) and EpiPen® to be available when the student is on the bus, whenever possible.
  Note: The EpiPen® should not remain on the bus overnight where it might be subject to temperature extremes.

- Arrangements for bus emergency protocols and procedures to include anaphylaxis.

- Facilitates a meeting between the bus driver and the child (and parents) prior to the start of school.

- Encourages the child with food allergies to always sit in a seat located towards the front of the bus.

- Institutes a strict "no eating" policy on the bus

- Makes sure that the bus's communication system is in good working order.

- Makes sure that the bus is cleaned regularly.

FOCUS AREA: SPECIAL PROGRAMMING

(Before/After School Events, Field Days, School Sports, Dances, School Drama Events, Teacher-Sponsored Events, etc.)

For all school sponsored events, regardless of whether these take place outside of normal school hours, precautions must be taken to keep the student with food allergies safe, and be consistent with the student's IHP. Coordination and cooperation between school personnel and the parent of the child with food allergies is critical to successful and safe programming. This means that:

- A staff member trained in EpiPen® administration should always be present for these events. This person may be the school nurse, but it could also be an EpiPen®-trained school staff member.

- The student's EpiPen® and related medications, and ETP must be present.

- Whenever possible, every effort should be made to eliminate the student's food allergens from being present at the event.

- A means of communication must be available, such as a cell phone, in order to access 911 should an allergic reaction occur.

- It is strongly recommended that the teacher communicate with the parent of the food-allergic student to inform them of the event and to make sure that all safety precautions have been considered and will be implemented.

FOCUS AREA: THE PLAYGROUND (ELEMENTARY LUNCH RECESS)

Lunch recess held outside presents risks to students with food allergies in a similar way to those found during gym class: there is physical interaction among students and play equipment used by the entire school community. Therefore:

- A school staff member assigned lunch aide duties will receive general food allergy education and training in EpiPen® administration by the school nurse. The school nurse will review the student's ETP with this lunch aide, as stated in the student's IHP.

- A medical bag containing the student's EpiPen® or EpiPen® Jr. and related medicines is carried by an EpiPen®-trained lunch aide assigned to the food-allergic student's lunch.

- The lunch aide is responsible for carrying a communication device, such as a cell phone or walkie-talkie, along with the medicine bag, to the playground during lunch recess.

- The school nurse will arrange for the lunch aide and the student to meet in order to facilitate visual recognition and help foster a comfortable relationship.

- A policy which requires that no food will be eaten on the playground after lunch, should be considered.

- In case of an allergic reaction, the lunch aide will notify the school health office and request that the nurse will respond. The lunch aide will remain with the child until the nurse arrives to treat the student. If symptoms escalate before the arrival of the nurse, the EpiPen®-trained lunch aide will administer the EpiPen®, according to the student's ETP.

- In the event that epinephrine is administered, 911 will be called, and the student will be transferred to the hospital. The student's parents will be promptly notified.

FOCUS AREA: THE EMERGENCY TREATMENT PLAN (ETP)

An Emergency Treatment Plan is a step-by-step plan for medical treatment and should be followed in the event a student experiences an allergic reaction. The plan is developed by the physician and should be reviewed thoroughly by the school nurse. It includes:

- The student's name and date of birth.

- A current, color photo of the student.

- The child's food allergies and related medical history.

- The signs and symptoms of an allergic reaction.

- Clear steps, in outline form, to treat the allergic reaction/ anaphylaxis.

- Emergency contact phone numbers for the parents and physician.

- The signature of the physician (a signature by the parent is also recommended).

FOCUS AREA: EVALUATION

An evaluation of a student's IHP is extremely important in making sure that the procedures within the IHP are both realistic and effective. It is recommended that an evaluation takes place:

- Whenever an allergic reaction occurs at school, so that changes may be made to reduce the likelihood of another one from happening.

- During late spring, so that the parents and the school nurse may plan for the subsequent school year. Changes/adjustments may be made to procedures within the student's IHP which will be consistent with the student's age and maturity.

MASTER CHECKLIST FOR AN IHP

FOCUS AREAS

Medical Documentation
Emergency Treatment Plan
Staff Training
- General Food Allergy Awareness
- EpiPen® Training

Educating the Student
The Classroom
- Materials Used
- Safe Snack Program
- Peer Education

Substitute Teachers
Substitute Nurses
"Specialist Teachers"
The Cafeteria
The Playground
- Classroom Recess
- Lunch Recess

Maintenance
Assemblies
Special Programming Events
- During the School Day
- Before or After School

Field Trips
School-wide Communication
Bus Transportation
Evaluation of IHP Procedures

INDIVIDUAL HEALTHCARE PLAN

IDENTIFYING INFORMATION

Student's Name: _____ School: _____

Date of Birth: _____ Teacher: _____

Age: _____ Principal: _____

Weight: _____ Nurse: _____

CONTACTS

PARENTS

Mother's Name: _____ Home Tel.: _____

Work Tel.: _____ Emergency Tel.: _____

Mother's Address: _____

Father's Name: _____ Home Tel.: _____

Work Tel.: _____ Emergency Tel.: _____

Father's Address: _____

PHYSICIAN

Physician/Allergist _____ Tel.: _____

Physician Address: _____

HOSPITAL

Hospital: _____ **Telephone:** _____

Hospital Address: _____

Ambulance Contact Telephone: _____

SCHOOL

School Nurse: _____ **Telephone:** _____

MEDICAL HISTORY

Medical Information: _____

Known Allergies: _____

Medications: _____

Related Health Concerns: _____

_____

INDIVIDUAL HEALTHCARE PLAN

STUDENT:
HOME PHONE:
D.O.B.:
SCHOOL: GRADE:
DATE OF IMPLEMENTATION:

STUDENT'S MEDICAL HISTORY:

GENERAL GOAL OF IHP:

Strict avoidance of allergens through risk reduction and avoidance accommodations. Plan for full inclusion.
_____ will not be segregated or isolated
    (Student Name)   from classroom curriculum.

RISKS (includes one or more of the following):

Exposure/Ingestion of allergen   Allergic reaction/Anaphylaxis
No EpiPen® trained staff   EpiPen® not readily accessible
Use of unsafe foods/materials   Segregation of student
No communication device when   Staff unaware of prevention
outside   protocols

Focus Area: THE PARENTS

Risk Reduction Steps: **Staff Responsible:**

1.

2.

3.

4.

5.

Focus Area: THE STUDENT

Risk Reduction Steps: **Staff Responsible:**

1.

2.

3.

4.

5.

Focus Area: HEALTH ROOM/NURSE

Risk Reduction Steps: **Staff Responsible:**

1.

2.

3.

4.

5.

Focus Area: SCHOOL ADMINISTRATION (Principal)

Risk Reduction Steps: **Staff Responsible:**

1.

2.

3.

4.

5.

Focus Area: THE CLASSROOM

Risk Reduction Steps: **Staff Responsible:**

1.

2.

3.

4.

5.

6.

7.

8.

9.

10.

11.

Focus Area: SUBSTITUTE TEACHERS

Risk Reduction Steps: **Staff Responsible:**

1.

2.

3.

4.

5.

6.

7.

Focus Area: SUBSTITUTE NURSE

Risk Reduction Steps: **Staff Responsible:**

1.

2.

3.

4.

5.

Focus Area: SPECIALISTS

<u>Risk Reduction Steps:</u>   **<u>Staff Responsible:</u>**

1.

2.

3.

4.

5.

Focus Area: FIELD TRIP

<u>Risk Reduction Steps:</u>   **<u>Staff Responsible:</u>**

1.

2.

3.

4.

5.

6.

7.

Focus Area: GYM

<u>Risk Reduction Steps:</u>   **<u>Staff Responsible:</u>**

1.

2.

3.

4.

5.

Focus Area: THE CAFETERIA

Risk Reduction Steps: **Staff Responsible:**

1.

2.

3.

4.

5.

Focus Area: BEFORE/AFTER SCHOOL EVENTS

Risk Reduction Steps: **Staff Responsible:**

1.

2.

3.

4.

5.

6.

7.

Focus Area: MAINTENANCE

Risk Reduction Steps: **Staff Responsible:**

1.

2.

3.

4.

5.

Focus Area: TRANSPORTATION

Risk Reduction Steps: **Staff Responsible:**

1.

2.

3.

4.

5.

6.

IHP has been reviewed and approved by:

_____   _____

School Nurse   Date

_____   _____

Principal   Date

_____   _____

Teacher   Date

_____   _____

Parents   Date

Anticipated Review Dates:

Attachments: **EMERGENCY TREATMENT PLAN**

Copyright © 2012 Educating For Food Allergies, LLC, All Rights Reserved

EMERGENCY TREATMENT PLAN (year)

Student Name: _____ **D.O.B.** _____

Teacher: _____ **Grade:** _____ **School:** _____

FOOD ALLERGY and MEDICAL HISTORY:

[Student Picture]

TREATMENT FOR ALLERGIC REACTION
MILD: Symptoms:

    Action: 1.)
             2.)
             3.)
             4.)
             5.)
             6.)

SEVERE or KNOWN INGESTION: Symptoms:

    Action: 1.)
             2.)
             3.)
             4.)
             5.)
             6.)

Parent Signature _____ Date: _____
Physician's Signature _____ Date: _____

EMERGENCY PHONE NUMBERS:

Name _____ Phone _____
Name _____ Phone _____
Allergist _____ Phone _____

©2012 Educating For Food Allergies, LLC

TRAINED STAFF MEMBERS:

Name: _____ Position: _____
Room# _____

Name: _____ Position: _____
Room# _____

Name: _____ Position: _____
Room# _____

DIRECTIONS FOR EPIPEN® and EPIPEN® JR.:

1.) Grasp EpiPen® auto-injector firmly in your fist. Orange Tip should point down.

2.) Pull off Blue Safety Release with other hand.

3.) Swing and firmly push Orange tip against outer thigh at 90 degree angle. *Hold and count slowly to 10.*

CALL 911

*You have received the correct dose of medication if the orange needle tip is extended and the window is obscured.

*Never put thumb, fingers or hand over the orange tip.

Copyright © 2012 *Educating for Food Allergies, LLC*

Food Allergy Action Plan
Emergency Care Plan

Name: _____ D.O.B.: ___ / ___ / ___

Allergy to: _____

Weight: _____ lbs.   **Asthma:** ☐ Yes (higher risk for a severe reaction)   ☐ No

Extremely reactive to the following foods: _____
THEREFORE:
☐ If checked, give epinephrine immediately for ANY symptoms if the allergen was *likely* eaten.
☐ If checked, give epinephrine immediately if the allergen was *definitely* eaten, even if no symptoms are noted.

Any SEVERE SYMPTOMS after suspected or known ingestion:	1. **INJECT EPINEPHRINE IMMEDIATELY**
One or more of the following:	2. Call 911
LUNG: Short of breath, wheeze, repetitive cough	3. Begin monitoring (see box below)
HEART: Pale, blue, faint, weak pulse, dizzy, confused	4. Give additional medications:* -Antihistamine -Inhaler (bronchodilator) if asthma
THROAT: Tight, hoarse, trouble breathing/swallowing	
MOUTH: Obstructive swelling (tongue and/or lips)	
SKIN: Many hives over body	*Antihistamines & inhalers/bronchodilators are not to be depended upon to treat a severe reaction (anaphylaxis). USE EPINEPHRINE.
Or **combination** of symptoms from different body areas:	
SKIN: Hives, itchy rashes, swelling (e.g., eyes, lips)	
GUT: Vomiting, diarrhea, crampy pain	

MILD SYMPTOMS ONLY:	1. **GIVE ANTIHISTAMINE**
MOUTH: Itchy mouth	2. Stay with student; alert healthcare professionals and parent
SKIN: A few hives around mouth/face, mild itch	3. If symptoms progress (see above), USE EPINEPHRINE
GUT: Mild nausea/discomfort	4. Begin monitoring (see box below)

Medications/Doses
Epinephrine (brand and dose): _____
Antihistamine (brand and dose): _____
Other (e.g., inhaler-bronchodilator if asthmatic): _____

Monitoring
Stay with student; alert healthcare professionals and parent. Tell rescue squad epinephrine was given; request an ambulance with epinephrine. Note time when epinephrine was administered. A second dose of epinephrine can be given 5 minutes or more after the first if symptoms persist or recur. For a severe reaction, consider keeping student lying on back with legs raised. Treat student even if parents cannot be reached. See back/attached for auto-injection technique.

_____   _____   _____   _____
Parent/Guardian Signature   Date   Physician/Healthcare Provider Signature   Date

TURN FORM OVER   Form provided courtesy of the Food Allergy & Anaphylaxis Network (www.foodallergy.org) 9/2011

Place Student's Picture Here

**EPIPEN Auto-Injector and
EPIPEN Jr Auto-Injector Directions**

- First, remove the EPIPEN Auto-Injector
  from the plastic carrying case

- **Pull off the blue safety release cap**

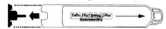

- **Hold orange tip near outer thigh
  (always apply to thigh)**

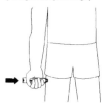

- **Swing and firmly push orange tip
  against outer thigh. Hold on thigh for
  approximately 10 seconds.
  Remove the EPIPEN Auto-Injector and
  massage the area for 10 more seconds**

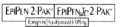

EPIPEN 2·PAK™ EPIPEN Jr 2·PAK™

[Epinephrine] Autoinjector 0.3 mg]

DEY™ and the Dey logo, EpiPen®, EpiPen 2·Pak®, and EpiPen Jr 2·Pak® are registered
trademarks of Dey Pharma, L.P.

Adrenaclick™ 0.3 mg and
Adrenaclick™ 0.15 mg Directions

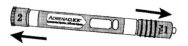

Remove GREY caps labeled
"1" and "2."

Place RED rounded tip against
outer thigh, press down hard until needle
penetrates. Hold for 10 seconds, then remove.

A food allergy response kit should
contain at least two doses of
epinephrine, other medications as
noted by the student's physician, and
a copy of this Food Allergy Action
Plan.

A kit must accompany the student if
he/she is off school grounds (i.e.,
field trip).

Contacts

Call 911 (Rescue squad: (___) _____-_____)   Doctor: _____   Phone: (___) _____-_____
Parent/Guardian: _____   Phone: (___) _____-_____

Other Emergency Contacts

Name/Relationship: _____   Phone: (___) _____-_____
Name/Relationship: _____   Phone: (___) _____-_____

Form provided courtesy of the Food Allergy & Anaphylaxis Network (www.foodallergy.org) 9/2011

Asthma and Allergy Foundation of America

The Food Allergy Network

EPA

CHILD CARE ASTHMA/ALLERGY ACTION CARD

ID Photo

Name: _____

Grade: _____ DOB: _____

Parent/Guardian Name: _____

Address: _____

Phone (H): _____ (W): _____

Parent/Guardian Name: _____

Address: _____

Phone (H): _____ (W): _____

Other Contact Information: _____

Emergency Phone Contact #1
Name _____

Relationship _____ Phone _____

Emergency Phone Contact #2
Name _____

Relationship _____ Phone _____

Physician Child Sees for Asthma/Allergies: _____

Phone: _____

Other Physician: _____

Phone: _____

- **Daily Medication Plan for Asthma/Allergy**

Name	Amount	When to Use
1		
2		
3		
4		

DAILY ASTHMA/ALLERGY MANAGEMENT PLAN

- **Identify the things that start an asthma/allergy episode**

  (Check each that applies to the child)

  — Animals   — Bee/Insect Sting   — Chalk Dust   — Change in Temperature

  — Dust Mites   — Exercise   — Latex   — Molds

  — Pollens   — Respiratory Infections   — Smoke   — Strong Odors

  — Food: _____

  — Other: _____

  Comments: _____

- **Peak Flow Monitoring** (for children over 4 years old)

  Personal Best Peak Flow reading: _____

  Monitoring Times: _____

- **Control of Child Care Environment** (List any environmental control measures, pre-medications, and/or dietary restrictions that the child needs to prevent an asthma/allergy episode.) _____

OUTSIDE ACTIVITY AND FIELD TRIPS The following medications must accompany child when participating in outside activity and field trips:

Name	Amount	When to Use
1		
2		
3		

ASTHMA EMERGENCY PLAN

Emergency action is necessary when the child has symptoms such as _____

or has a peak flow reading at or below. _____

- **Steps to take during an asthma episode:**

1. Check peak flow reading (if child uses a peak flow meter).
2. Give medications as listed below.
3. Check for decreased symptoms and/or increased peak flow reading.
4. Allow child to stay at child care setting if: _____

5. Contact parent/guardian

6. Seek emergency medical care if the child has any one of the following:

→ No improvement minutes after initial treatment with medication.
→ Peak flow at or below _____
→ Hard time breathing with:
   ➤ Chest and neck pulled in with breathing.
   ➤ Child hunched over.
   ➤ Child struggling to breathe.
→ Trouble walking or talking.
→ Stops playing and cannot start activity again.
→ Lips or fingernails are gray or blue.

IF THIS HAPPENS, GET EMERGENCY HELP NOW! →

- **Emergency Asthma Medications:**

	Name	Amount	When to Use
1			
2			
3			
4			

- **Special Instructions:**

Physician's Signature	Date	Parent/Guardian's Signature	Date

ALLERGY EMERGENCY PLAN

- **Child is allergic to:** _____

- **Steps to take during an allergy episode:**

1. If the following symptoms occur, give the medications listed below.
2. Contact Emergency help and request epinephrine.
3. Contact the child's parent/guardian

- **Symptoms of an allergic reaction include:**

(Physician, please circle those that apply)

→ **Mouth/Throat:** itching & swelling of lips, tongue, mouth, throat; throat tightness, hoarseness, cough
→ **Skin:** hives; itchy rash; swelling
→ **Gut:** nausea; abdominal cramps; vomiting; diarrhea
→ **Lung*:** shortness of breath; coughing; wheezing
→ **Heart*:** pulse is hard to detect; "passing out"
*If child has asthma, asthma symptoms may also need to be treated.

- **Emergency Allergy Medications:**

	Name	Amount	When to Use
1			
2			
3			
4			

- **Special Instructions:**

Child Care Provider's Signature	Date

*Source: Asthma and Allergy Foundation of America, www.aafa.org

Student Name _____

D.O.B. _____

School _____

Date _____

WORKSHEET FOR INDIVIDUAL HEALTHCARE PLAN

FOCUS AREA	RISKS	RISK REDUCTION PLAN OF ACTION	STAFF RESPONSIBLE FOR IMPLEMENTATION
1. Educating the Student			
2. Staff Training			
3. The Classroom			

STUDENT NAME

FOCUS AREA	RISKS	RISK REDUCTION PLAN OF ACTION	STAFF RESPONSIBLE FOR IMPLEMENTATION
4. SUBSTITUTE TEACHERS			
5. SUBSTITUTE NURSES			
6. SPECIALISTS			

STUDENT NAME			
FOCUS AREA	RISKS	RISK REDUCTION PLAN OF ACTION	STAFF RESPONSIBLE FOR IMPLEMENTATION
7. THE CAFETERIA			
8. THE PLAYGROUND			
9. MAINTENANCE			

STUDENT NAME			
FOCUS AREA	RISKS	RISK REDUCTION PLAN OF ACTION	STAFF RESPONSIBLE FOR IMPLEMENTATION
10. ASSEMBLIES			
11. SPECIAL PROGRAMMING			
12. FIELD TRIPS			

STUDENT NAME			
FOCUS AREA	RISKS	RISK REDUCTION PLAN OF ACTION	STAFF RESPONSIBLE FOR IMPLEMENTATION
13. SCHOOL-WIDE COMMUNICATION			
14. BUS TRANSPORTATION			
15. EVALUATION			

STUDENT NAME			
FOCUS AREA	RISKS	RISK REDUCTION PLAN OF ACTION	STAFF RESPONSIBLE FOR IMPLEMENTATION
16. EMERGENCY TREATMENT PLAN (ETP)			

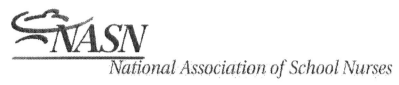

Position Statement
Individualized Healthcare Plans (IHP)

SUMMARY OF THE POSITION:

It is the position of the National Association of School Nurses (NASN) that students whose healthcare needs affect or have the potential to affect safe and optimal school attendance and academic performance require the professional school nurse to write an Individualized Healthcare Plan (IHP), in collaboration with the student, family, educators, and healthcare care providers. It is also the position of NASN that it is the responsibility of the professional school nurse to implement and evaluate the IHP at least yearly to determine the need for revision and evidence of desired student outcomes.

HISTORY:

The IHP is a written document that outlines the provision of student healthcare services intended to achieve specific student outcomes. The management of school healthcare services for students with significant or chronic health problems is a vital role for school nurses (National Association of School Nurses [NASN] & American Nurses Association [ANA], 2005). The standard for this role is based on the nursing process and must include: Assessment, Nursing Diagnosis, Outcome Identification, Planning, Implementation, and Evaluation. Documentation of these steps for individual students who have healthcare issues results in the development of Individualized Healthcare Plans (IHPs), a variation of nursing care plans. IHPs fulfill administrative and clinical purposes including management of healthcare conditions to promote learning; facilitating communication, coordination, and continuity of care among service providers; and evaluation/revision of care provided (Herrmann, 2005).

DESCRIPTION OF ISSUE:

Chronic mental and physical health conditions or disabilities can interfere with school participation and achievement. Many students with stable conditions, such as attention deficit-hyperactivity or mild intermittent asthma, require basic school nursing services such as health care monitoring or medication administration. Some students need specialized services and require an IHP, which may include an emergency care plan (ECP) and/or a field trip plan. The need for an IHP is based on required nursing care, not educational entitlement such as special education or Section 504 of the Rehabilitation Act of 1973.

Sometimes, students need the additional protections of federal laws in order to fully participate in an educational program. PL 93-112 Section 504 of the Rehabilitation Act of 1973 (also called Section 504) identifies criteria that indicate accommodations may be required (504 plan) for an eligible student. PL 108-446 (2004), the Individuals with Disabilities Education Improvement Act (IDEIA) entitles students who are eligible for special education to receive services that are necessary to access or benefit from their educational program. Special healthcare services are outlined in the Individual Education Plan (IEP). For special education students, the IHP may be included as an attachment to the IEP.

The nursing process "provides the framework for the delivery and evaluation of nursing care" to students (Denehy, 2004, p. 7). *The Scope and Standards of Practice* (NASN & ANA, 2005) outlines how each step of the

National Association of School Nurses, Inc.
8484 Georgia Avenue
Suite 420
Silver Spring, Maryland 20910

1-240-821-1130
1-301-585-1791 Fax
http://www.nasn.org
nasn@nasn.org

nursing process is implemented to strengthen and facilitate educational outcomes for students. These steps parallel components of a well-written IHP.

Standard 1. Assessment: The data collection phase helps determine the student's current health status and any actual or potential health concerns.
Standard 2. Diagnosis: The professional school nurse uses the assessment data to formulate a nursing diagnosis, including a diagnostic label, etiology, and presenting signs and symptoms.
Standard 3. Outcome Identification: The professional school nurse identifies the desired results of nursing intervention and states these in measurable terms.
Standard 4. Planning: Interventions are selected to achieve desired results.
Standard 5. Implementation: The written IHP is put into practice and care provided is documented.
Standard 6. Evaluation: The professional school nurse measures the effectiveness of nursing interventions in meeting the identified outcome. Changes are made to the plan as needed.

The school nurse must determine which students require an IHP, prioritizing those students whose healthcare needs affect their daily functioning or safety. These students may have multiple healthcare needs, require lengthy procedures or treatments, require routine or emergency contact with the school nurse or unlicensed assistive personnel during the school day, or require special healthcare services as part of their IEP or Section 504 plan.

Performance and documentation of the nursing process are professional school nursing functions that cannot be delegated (National Council of State Boards of Nursing, 2005). The registered professional school nurse is responsible and accountable for creating the individualized healthcare plan (IHP), for managing its activities, and for its outcomes, even when implementation of the plan requires delegation to unlicensed assistive personnel (NASNa, 2006).

The IHP is developed collaboratively with information from the family, the student, the student's healthcare providers, and school staff, as appropriate (NASN & ANA, 2005). The IHP includes medical orders implemented at school. Evaluation identifies progress toward achieving student outcomes. The IHP is reviewed at least annually, updated as needed, and revised as significant changes occur in the student's health status or medical treatment.

Standardized IHP's, printed or computerized, are available for common chronic pediatric health conditions. These standardized plans help promote continuity of care but individualization is essential in order to meet the unique needs of each student. In addition, NASN encourages the use of standardized language such as North American Nursing Diagnosis Association-International (NANDA), Nursing Interventions Classification (NIC) and Nursing Outcomes Classification (NOC) in IHP development (Denehy, 2004). Standardized language facilitates communication with other nursing staff and data collection, links student health care and education outcomes, and helps nurses evaluate correlations between interventions and outcomes (NASNb, 2006). Furthermore, the use of standardized language enhances development of a common knowledge base for school nursing which is essential for evidence-based practice (Poulton and Denehy, 2005).

RATIONALE:

Professional school nurses are leaders in the provision of special healthcare services. Through coordination of care among the school and the home, primary and specialty medical care, and clinics, school nurses ensure continuity of care across settings and minimize the risk for miscommunication (Taras et al., 2004). School nurses are also responsible for the training, direction, and supervision of both licensed and unlicensed personnel and the delegation of select nursing tasks as directed by individual state nurse practice acts (NASN & ANA, 2005). An IHP is the written document that captures these professional activities provided to individual students (Selekman, 2006).

National Association of School Nurses, Inc.
8484 Georgia Avenue
Suite 420
Silver Spring, Maryland 20910

1-240-821-1130
1-301-585-1791 Fax
http://www.nasn.org
nasn@nasn.org

References/Resources

Denehy, J. (2004). *Using nursing languages in school nursing practice.* Silver Spring, MD: National Association of School Nurses.

Herrmann, D. (2005). Individualized healthcare plans. In C. Silkworth, M. Arnold, J. Harrigan, & D. Zaiger, (Eds.) *Individualized healthcare plans for the school nurse. pp. 1-5.* North Branch, MN: Sunrise River Press.

National Association of School Nurses. (2004). Position statement: *Emergency care plans for students with special health care needs.* Retrieved from http://www.nasn.org/Default.aspx?tabid=220.

National Association of School Nurses. (2006a). Position statement: *Standardized nursing languages.* Available at http://www.nasn.org/Default.aspx?tabid=233.

National Association of School Nurses. (2006b). Position statement: *School nursing management of students with chronic health conditions.* Retrieved from http://www.nasn.org/Default.aspx?tabid=351.

National Association of School Nurses & American Nurses Association. (2005). *School nursing: Scope and standards of practice.* Silver Spring, MD: NursesBooks.Org.

National Council of State Boards of Nursing. (2005). *Working with others: A position paper.* Chicago, IL. Author.

Poulton, S. & Denehy, J. (2005). Integrating NANDA, NIC, and NOC into individualized healthcare plans. In C. Silkworth, M. Arnold, J. Harrigan, & D. Zaiger (Eds.) *Individualized healthcare plans for the school nurse (pp. 25-36).* North Branch, MN: Sunrise River Press.

Rehabilitation Act of 1973, 29 U.S.C. 794 § 504; regulations at 34 C.F.R. pt. 104 (1973).

Selekman, J. (Ed.). (2006). *School nursing: A comprehensive text.* Philadelphia, PA: F.A. Davis Company.

Taras, H., Duncan, P., Luckenbill, D., Robinson, J., Wheeler, L., & Wooley, S. (2004). *Health, mental health and safety guidelines for schools.* Retrieved from, http://www.nationalguidelines.org.

Adopted: June 1998
Revised: November 2003; March 2008; June 2008

National Association of School Nurses, Inc
8484 Georgia Avenue
Suite 420
Silver Spring, Maryland 20910

1-240-821-1130
1-301-585-1791 Fax
http://www.nasn.org
nasn@nasn.org

INDIVIDUAL HEALTHCARE PLAN (IHP)
VS. 504 PLAN

DIFFERENCES:

A **504 plan** is a <u>legal document</u> which is a product of *Section 504 of the Rehabilitation Act of 1973*. In order to determine a student's eligibility for 504 protection, a formal process which includes an evaluation meeting should take place. Medical documentation from the student's physician of the diagnosis of a life-threatening allergy should be provided.

An **IHP** is considered a documented plan of care. An **IHP** does not require a *formal* evaluation meeting. Schools may require documentation from a physician which verifies the child's allergy.

A **504 Plan** denotes legal accountability from the beginning, which means staff is legally responsible for implementation of its accommodations as written.

It is a reasonable expectation that an **IHP**, once agreed upon, will designate staff responsible for implementation of its procedures as written.

The **504 coordinator** is considered head of the core team for a **504 Plan**, but is not usually considered part of the core team for an **IHP**. The **school nurse** is responsible for planning appropriate accommodations within the student's **504 Plan**. Input from the parents is important, but not legally required.

For an **IHP**, the school nurse is considered the coordinator of the core team, and is responsible, with help from the parents, to plan appropriate procedures.

For a **504 Plan**, the parents are not legally required to be members of the core team, however it is considered best practice.

For an **IHP**, parents should be considered an integral part of the core team.

For a **504 Plan**, there is a formal grievance procedure.

For an **IHP**, there is no formal grievance procedure.

SIMILARITIES:

For a **504 Plan** and an **IHP**, accommodations will be similar, if not the same.

For a **504 Plan** and an **IHP**, the parent's signature is <u>not required</u> but is considered best practice.

Both **504 Plans** and **IHPs** can help to insure that modifications and accommodations are made to the school program to enhance a food-allergic student's safety while at school.

FOOD-FREE BIRTHDAY CELEBRATIONS !!!

☺ Birthday child selects book to donate to the library. His/her name (and picture) goes in the front of the book.

☺ Birthday child shares a special item with classmates (e.g. favorite book, favorite song, favorite stuffed animal, favorite picture or souvenir, etc.).

☺ Birthday child chooses a game that classmates will play during recess.

☺ Birthday child is the classroom "leader" for the day (e.g. morning meeting, Pledge of Allegiance, line to cafeteria).

☺ Classmates design and decorate a Birthday crown to be worn by the Birthday child.

☺ Classmates each prepare a page about the Birthday child; teacher compiles pages and then reads "book" to the class.

☺ Birthday child wears a special button for the day.

☺ Birthday child invites a special visitor to the class to read a story.

☺ Birthday child brings in photos of his/her life, and explains each picture.

☺ Birthday child brings in special party "gifts" to share with classmates (e.g. stickers, pencils, erasers, notepads, etc.).

☺ Birthday child's name is announced over the school PA system or at "All School Meeting"

☺ Birthday child's name is announced at lunch in the cafeteria, and everyone sings "Happy Birthday To You".

☺ Birthday child and friends eat lunch with the teacher in the cafeteria.

Copyright © 2012 *Educating For Food Allergies, LLC* All Rights Reserved

Sample School Letter

Date:

Dear Parents:

This school year, your child will be in the same classroom as a student who has a life threatening allergy to peanuts and nuts. As a result, the following information is meant to help you plan for the coming year.

It is important to understand that even a small amount of the food to which a child is allergic can cause that child to have a serious allergic reaction. In fact, a fatal reaction can occur after eating as little as 1/250 of a peanut. Exposure from cross-contamination is also an issue with food allergies. A child may develop an allergic reaction by merely touching a surface on which there is peanut residue. Therefore, certain procedures will be put into place to ensure the safety of all students in the classroom, and allow the primary focus to be on learning.

The classroom will be designated as peanut/nut free, and as such, we are requesting that you do not send in any snacks which contain peanuts, nuts or peanut butter. We would appreciate it if you would alert your child of the potential dangers to his/her classmates if products of this nature are brought to school. If your child eats any of these foods for breakfast, we also ask that you have your child's hands washed and teeth brushed before coming to school.

There will be a plan for safe foods used for holidays and birthday celebrations this year. The specific details for this will be explained in the letter you will receive from your child's teacher. In addition, your child may be asked to sit at a peanut-free table at some point during the school year. If you are notified that your child has been asked to sit at this table, please remember to not send in any peanut/nut products at that time. If you have any concerns about the possibility of your child sitting at this table, please let the teacher know at the start of the school year.

Your support for these important safety precautions is greatly appreciated and we thank you in advance for your cooperation. Please sign your name on the form below, and return it to the school nurse. If you have any questions, please contact either the school nurse or principal.

Sincerely,

_____   _____

School Nurse   School Principal

Please tear off and return to the school nurse

I have read and understand the peanut/nut free classroom procedures, and I will cooperate with these procedures to help keep the room safe for all students.

Child's Name: _____

Classroom Teacher's Name: _____

Parent Signature: _____

Date: _____

IMPORTANT NOTICE TO ALL TEACHERS AND STAFF:

FOOD ALLERGIES AT THE HOLIDAY SEASON

As we look forward to the holiday season, we realize that it is sometimes the practice of teachers and staff to hand out "treats" to the students. We would like to encourage you to share non-food treats at this time. If you are considering sharing food treats with your students, please remember that there are children at school with severe food allergies.

Before any food items are handed out, please check all the ingredients with the school nurse. ***Please do not assume that a food is safe; all ingredients listed on candies and treats need to be read.***

Your cooperation with this protocol is critical to the safety of children at school with severe food allergies. We wish everyone a healthy and joyous holiday season.

END-OF-THE-YEAR PARTIES:
FOOD ALLERGY REMINDER!

TO ALL TEACHERS AND STAFF:

As the end of the year draws near, some of you may be planning end-of-the-year parties. If any of your plans involve food as part of the festivities, it is critical that certain procedures be followed in classes which have students with food allergies.

Please contact the school nurse so that the food(s) you are planning to serve, and their ingredients, can be discussed to determine that they are allergen-free. *It is very important that no assumptions be made regarding whether a food is safe*. The school nurse will be able to give you as much assistance in this area as you need.

Your cooperation is critical for the safety of the children and is greatly appreciated by their parents.

Thank you.

Name of School: _____

<u>Substitute Teacher Checklist:</u>

Substitute teachers will be called by: _____.

When a substitute is called for the following teachers:

(names of teachers who have a student(s) in their classroom with a food allergy)

The caller will notify the substitute teacher that they must report to the school nurse before going into the classroom. The school nurse will review the following information with the Substitute Teacher:

1. The student's Individual Healthcare Plan

2. The student's Emergency Treatment Plan

3. Symptoms of an allergic reaction and anaphylaxis

4. The snack program/cafeteria procedures

5. <u>**NO**</u> food or snacks should be handed out (unless approved by the school nurse/parent)

LIST OF STATES WITH GUIDELINES FOR SCHOOL FOOD ALLERGY MANAGEMENT
as of May, 2012

Alabama—NO.

Alaska—NO.

Arizona—YES: "Arizona Resource Guide for Supporting Children with Life-Threatening Food Allergies"

Arkansas—NO.

California—NO. (The California State PTA is calling for the development and implementation of state guidelines.)

Colorado—Senate Bill 226 was signed into law by Governor Ritter and requires the State Board of Education, in conjunction with the State Department of Public Health and Environment, to put into effect food allergy and anaphylaxis management rules for public school districts. The State Charter School Institute will be required to do the same with charter schools.

Connecticut—YES: "Guidelines for Managing Life-Threatening Food Allergies in Connecticut Schools"

Delaware—NO.

Florida—NO. "Florida School District Food Allergy Policies" is a report issued by Florida Department of Education Commissioner, Eric Smith to Florida Governor Crist and the Florida Legislature, December 31, 2009. Report states the value in developing statewide guidelines.

Georgia—NO.

Hawaii—NO.

Idaho—NO.

Illinois—YES: "Guidelines for Managing Life-Threatening Food Allergies in Illinois Schools". Policies based on these guidelines to be implemented by school boards by January 1, 2011.

Indiana—NO.

Iowa—NO.

Kansas—NO. House Bill 2008 was approved by the Governor; it states that accredited schools may obtain epinephrine kits from licensed pharmacists and keep these kits at school to use in the event of anaphylaxis.

Kentucky—NO.

Louisiana—NO.

Maine—NO. The Maine Department of Education, School Health Manual, states that for allergies, it is the role of the nurse to establish 504 Plans as needed, and that an Individual Health Plan and an Emergency Plan should be prepared for students with severe allergies. The Manual calls on school nurses to develop school guidelines for students with food allergies.

Maryland—YES: "Management of Students at Risk for Anaphylactic Reaction", 2009.

Massachusetts—YES: "Managing Life Threatening Food Allergies in Schools", 2002.

Michigan—NO. Senate Bill 233 was introduced on February 17, 2009 and calls for the adoption and implementation of a policy for pupils with serious food allergies.

Minnesota—NO.

Mississippi—YES: "Managing Food Allergies in Mississippi Schools—Guidelines", 2008.

Missouri—YES: "Guidelines for Allergy Prevention and Response", 2012.

Montana—NO.

Nebraska—NO. Legislative Bill 72, introduced on January 8, 2009, would have called for policy guidelines to be provided which address the management of students with life threatening allergies. It failed to advance with a vote of 21-27.

Nevada—NO.

New Hampshire—NO.

New Jersey—YES: "Guidelines for the Management of Life-Threatening Food Allergies in Schools", 2008.

New Mexico—NO.

New York—YES: "Caring for Students with Life Threatening Allergies", 2007.

North Carolina—NO.

North Dakota—NO.

Ohio—YES: Ohio Revised Code Section 3313.719, per House Bill 1, dated July, 2009, requires written policy to protect students with peanut or other food allergies.

Oklahoma—NO.

Oregon—NO.

Pennsylvania—YES: "Pennsylvania Guidelines for Management of Food Allergies in Schools", 2011.

Rhode Island—NO. School food allergy management regulation: RI General Laws 16-21-SCHO, Section 18.11-18.17. (peanut/tree nut allergies, specifically addressed.)

South Carolina—NO.

South Dakota—NO.

Tennessee—YES: "2007 Guidelines for Use of Health Care Professionals and Health Care Procedures in a School Setting", includes Guidelines for Managing Life-Threatening Food Allergies.

Texas—YES: Senate Bill 27 requires statewide food allergy management guidelines to be created for Texas schools by August 1, 2012.

Utah—NO.

Vermont—YES: "Managing Life-Threatening Allergic Conditions in Schools", 2008.

Virginia—NO.

Washington—YES: "Guidelines for Care of Students with Anaphylaxis", 2009.

West Virginia—YES: "West Virginia Department of Education Guidelines for Allergies in the School Setting".

Wisconsin—YES, with limitations: "Guidelines for Managing Life Threatening Food Allergies in Schools." Addresses special dietary needs, safety precautions for food preparation and handling and food on field trips. Does not address risk reduction for the classroom.

(Prepared by the Wisconsin Department of Public Instruction, School Nutrition Team)

Wyoming—NO.

*Check with your state department of education for updated information

"Patience and fortitude conquer all things."

Ralph Waldo Emerson

CHAPTER THREE

THE NEED FOR SCHOOL DISTRICT LIFE-THREATENING FOOD ALLERGY POLICIES

A review of the literature and studies stated in previous chapters provides a clear overview of the serious nature of food allergies. The number of students with life-threatening food allergies attending schools today is growing at an increasingly alarming rate. Equally alarming is the fact that every food-allergic reaction has the potential to develop into anaphylaxis and that anaphylaxis itself may occur within minutes of exposure to the offending allergen. In addition, we know that the school setting presents a particularly high risk environment for students with food allergies. School personnel have a responsibility to provide a **safe environment for *all* students**, including their student population with food allergies.

Need for Consistency

In my experience, it is not unusual to find inconsistencies in the ways in which each school within a district addresses food allergy management. For example, some schools within a district may have sound procedures and protocols in place for their food-allergic students, while other schools within that same district have programs which are significantly different and even insufficient by comparison. To complicate matters even more, there may also be schools within the same district that have nothing at all in place to address food allergy management. This scenario can create understandable confusion and even resentment when a family with a food-allergic child lives in an area in which the assigned school does not have adequate risk-reduction practices in place. This often becomes a catalyst for parents who wish to move their child to a school "out of district" and out of their neighborhood in order to enroll their son or daughter at a school that seems to "get it". Accomplishing the task of switching schools may be a complicated and lengthy process, and, in some cases, is simply not allowed. As a result, dissatisfaction and conflict may result and cause real problems for both parents and school administration alike. Confusion and discord caused for these reasons are not only unnecessary and undesirable, but are avoidable.

School administrators must set as a priority the development of district policy for the management of food allergies and anaphylaxis. The foundation of this policy and the protocols and procedures within it must be standardized to ensure consistency in its interpretation and in its implementation throughout the school district. In addition, the goals of a food allergy management policy should be to 1.) have a system in place to identify all students with life-threatening food allergies, 2.) minimize the risk of allergic reactions in children with life-threatening food allergies while they are at school and while participating in school-sponsored events, 3.) educate school personnel to recognize the symptoms of an allergic reaction and 4.) train staff to be competent to administer emergency procedures in accordance with the student's emergency treatment plan. It is also critical that the policy address specific protocols to follow if anaphylaxis were to occur in a previously undiagnosed individual. This would require authorization by the school physician to write standing orders for epinephrine to be administered by the school nurse in the case of such an emergency. The policy must also include protocols which address the circumstances under which a student would be allowed to carry and administer their own Epinephrine auto-injector.

LIFE THREATENING ALLERGY DISTRICT POLICY
A PARENT'S PERSPECTIVE

When our daughter with life threatening allergies to peanuts, tree nuts and sesame, as well as asthma, began kindergarten 6 years ago, we were like most parents of food allergic kids, quite nervous. We made plans to speak with the school principal the spring before our daughter was due to start kindergarten. We were shocked and surprised, and angry, about the responses we received from that principal on how she intended to manage allergies at school. At the time, our school district had no district policy on life threatening allergies, and decisions were left to the discretion of each school's principal. This meant that how each student's allergies were managed could vary greatly from school to school, and even student to student within the same school. This principal was very rigid and unwilling to make required accommodations for our daughter. She even refused to use the language "life threatening" when referring to her allergies. She said that she could not make special considerations for our daughter, because it would impose on the rights of the other students at the school.

The district policy was a hard fought struggle to make the importance of food allergies and the importance of a policy to guide school employees come to full light. It took almost 2 years, but since the time when a policy was finalized in our school district, life threatening allergies now receives the attention they deserve and we are no longer looked at as "the annoying" parents looking for accommodations for our daughter's safety and wellbeing at school. The policy has made the school accountable to meet a standard in addressing life threatening allergies appropriately, regardless of which school a student with food allergies attends in town. The district policy not only leveled the playing field across the district, it has given the schools a place to continue the discussion on an ongoing basis. Our Wellness Committee has a sub-committee dedicated to life threatening allergies and several times per year this sub-committee reviews the policy and makes recommendations as necessary for improvements or changes.

Our daughter is now heading to the middle school next year. As parents of a child with life threatening allergies, we will again be nervous with this change. Yet, because of the strides made in our schools as a result of the adoption of a district wide life threatening allergy policy, we will know that our questions and concerns will be taken seriously and that school administration will work with us for the goal of our daughter's safety and wellbeing.

Fiona Murphy, Parent
Walpole, Massachusetts

The Process for Establishing a District Policy

The procedure to develop and establish any written school policy requires many steps before it may become adopted and ultimately implemented within a school system. As with any new idea or objective, it usually takes one person to start the process. It should not matter whether this enlightened individual is a parent, a school nurse, the principal or the Superintendent. What does matter is that someone with a position of authority listens. Realistically, it requires that someone who has a professional position within the school district administration either initiates or responds to the request that a district-wide policy on food allergies be considered and constructed.

The best way to start this process would be to establish a planning committee. In order to optimize the functioning and productivity of the committee, it is important that a leader be designated so that all proceedings will be coordinated in a comprehensive and systematic way. Once the committee has been formed, there should be meetings scheduled on a regular basis. Every member of the planning committee should be considered an integral part of this effort and should be assigned a role and/or task. In addition, a committee member should be assigned the responsibility of taking the notes for each meeting, which should then be transcribed, copied and distributed at each subsequent meeting. This facilitates a continuing thread of content and thought and allows for important points previously made not to be forgotten.

As progress is made and goals are defined, a rough draft of the district policy should be developed. When the committee is ready to make this draft public, a request should be made to the School Committee for space to be put on the agenda for its presentation. Inclusion on the agenda of a public School Committee meeting will mean questions and discussion from members of the School Committee, but also from interested members of the community. Comments will undoubtedly run the gamut from requests for clarification to statements of both support and opposition. It is possible for the document to be sent back to the planning committee for further development several times before it is ultimately agreed upon and adopted as policy by the School Committee. Because of the level and degree of work required, it is not uncommon for this entire process to take a full year.

Who should comprise the membership of this planning committee? It is strongly recommended that members of the committee represent a collaboration of all parties who have a vested interest in the outcome of the written policy. Therefore, members of this planning committee should include, but are not limited to the Superintendent or his/her designee, the school administrative staff member responsible for students with special needs (often referred to as the Director of Student Services), the district nurse leader, a school principal, a teacher and a small number of parents of children with food allergies (one to three parents will usually allow for a balanced representation of ideas and perspectives). Additional personnel considered for participation on this committee would be the Director of Food Services and the Director of Bus Transportation.

LIFE THREATENING ALLERGY DISTRICT POLICY: A SCHOOL ADMINISTRATOR'S PERSPECTIVE

The Canton Public Schools needed to reevaluate its allergy policy primarily due to the use of food in the curriculum and within the school for celebrations and rewards. Due to the increasing numbers of students with allergies to various types of foods, we felt it was prudent to revisit this policy to ensure that it protected the safety and welfare of our students and staff and yet still allowed for limited use of food in the curriculum and in school celebrations where warranted. We developed a committee representative of the school constituencies including teachers, parents, administrators and nurses. The end result of our year long work is a food allergy policy which ensured a safe learning environment for students and staff with limitations on how and when food may be used for teaching and celebration.

Alan B. Dewey, Assistant Superintendent for Student Services, Canton Public Schools, Massachusetts

Suggested Publications to Reference for District Policy Development

As the committee begins the task of drafting its district policy on food allergy management, it is important to understand that language used must have a clear message of intent and purpose. At the same time, the policy language should not be so rigid that it does not allow for the implementation of procedures which meet each student's individual needs. Given these requirements, great care must be taken to insure that the final product is thoughtfully written, carefully constructed and comprehensive. While it is certain that extensive research should be conducted, there are at least four important publications which should be referenced for this process. Specifically, they are:

- *"Managing Life Threatening Food Allergies in Schools"*—Guidelines produced by the Massachusetts Department of Elementary and Secondary Education.

- *"Anaphylaxis in Schools and Other Childcare Settings"*—1998 Position Statement offered by the American Academy of Allergy, Asthma, and Immunology (AAAAI).

- *"Individualized Healthcare Plans (IHP)"*—2008 Position Statement from the National Association of School Nurses (NASN).

- *"Accommodating Children with Special Dietary Needs in the School Nutrition Programs"*—United States Department of Agriculture, Food and Nutrition Service guidance manual for school food service staff.

These documents offer professional advice, broad-based recommendations and clear guidance for managing food allergies at school. Consultation with these and other similar publications will assist the district in writing protocols which are consistent with established standards of care.

An important consideration would be to reference and link aspects of the district's Wellness Policy, if one exists, to the Life Threatening

Allergy (LTA) Policy. For example, protocols within a district food allergy policy might include prohibiting the use of candy and other high sugar/fat foods as part of a reward system by the teacher in the classroom. Similarly, there also may be protocols which suggest or require that non-food activities are enjoyed when celebrating birthdays, as an alternative to having cake and ice cream, for example. Although offered in a food allergy policy as a way to reduce food-allergic reactions, these same protocols may be found in a Wellness Policy as a means of addressing the growing incidence of diabetes and obesity in school-aged children. When the same procedures are effective as a means to address several health concerns, it lends to the importance of their inclusion in both district policies.

Communication of District Policy to the School Community

Another area to address in the district policy would be the requirement for the district policy to be communicated to the school community. Inclusion of suggestions for ways in which to accomplish this are also recommended. Examples might be sharing pertinent policy information in letters sent by the school principal and/or school nurse to all families within the school community. This could be done at the beginning of the school year and then again at high risk times such as during the holidays. Topics covered might include a general explanation of food allergies and anaphylaxis offered as a means of education, along with the request for assistance in helping to keep students with food allergies in the school community safe. Other means of effective communication might be through letters sent by the classroom teacher to all parents of families in the classroom which describe more specific food allergen procedures in place, including an explanation of why they have been instituted. Many schools have utilized the school's Student Handbook as a medium to present the school's policy and procedures regarding food allergy management.

Topics covered in this communication could include information on signs located within the school which post allergy protocols, procedures to be followed whenever a bake sale is to be held, possible restrictions on food consumption outside of the classroom and cafeteria, prohibiting the sale of certain foods, hand washing procedures being implemented at the school, etc. Kindergarten orientation is also an opportune time to introduce families to food allergy protocols in place at the school and their role in supporting these procedures. Actively communicating the district's food allergy policy and related procedures will serve to enhance the school community's awareness and understanding of this issue and how it will be handled.

Compliance with Federal and State Laws and Regulations

District policy must address and comply with all federal and state laws which protect the rights of children with life-threatening food allergies, such as Section 504 of the Rehabilitation Act of 1973, the Americans with Disabilities Act of 1990, and the Individuals with Disabilities Education Act. These laws were written to ensure that individuals with disabilities will not be discriminated against or isolated in any way, and will, in fact, benefit from the same rights and privileges as individuals without disabilities. Because Section 504 of the Rehabilitation Act specifically recognizes allergy as a "hidden disability", it is appropriate for district policy on food allergy to reference 504 Plans as a viable means of managing a student's food allergies.

Another federal law which must be referenced in the policy is USDA Federal Regulation - 7 CFR, 15b, which addresses the School Breakfast Program and the National School Lunch Program. This regulation explains the responsibility of the school's food service department in providing meals for students who are considered to have a disability. Policy language must make clear these requirements and expectations for school administrators and nutrition staff to follow. Additional state regulations, such as those that govern nursing practices should also be reviewed and referenced in the policy. For example, each state has regulations regarding the administration of medications which must be followed. The procedures outlined in the district policy must be consistent with these legal requirements. The district may also wish to reference the state's Good Samaritan law which does not hold school employees liable should they, in good faith, respond to a medical emergency. Another issue which must be addressed in the policy is the right to confidentiality for the student with food allergies. This must be made clear through a presentation of the requirements found in the Family Educational Rights and Privacy Act (FERPA) and the Health Insurance Portability and Accountability Act of 1966 (HIPAA). Thoughtful planning and consideration of all applicable laws and regulations when writing district policy will not only enable the district to lessen the likelihood of liability issues, but will also help to lessen the risk of anaphylaxis for these students who have special healthcare needs.

Policy Format

A district policy template should include four basic areas: a *Policy Statement, Background Information, Purpose and Goal* of the policy and *Procedures* to be followed within that policy. The "Policy Statement" section gives an overview of the intention of the policy to address food allergy management within the school system. The "Background Information" section explains the nature of food allergies and anaphylaxis, highlighting the need for a comprehensive policy to be in place as a means to adequately address this medical concern. The "Purpose and Goal" section states in clear terms the expected outcome of the written policy. The "Procedures" section is a particularly important component to the policy because it gives specific guidance and directives to school staff as to their roles and responsibilities in order to support the purpose and goals of the policy. References to sources should be given explicitly in the event that additional information is desired, and all support documents referenced in the policy should be incorporated into the appendix. In addition, a glossary added at the back of the policy is recommended in order to facilitate a clear understanding of terminology used throughout the policy, such as "anaphylaxis", "epinephrine", Individual Healthcare Plan".

In conclusion, when a carefully constructed district policy on food allergy management is put in writing and adopted, it demonstrates a strong and official commitment by the district to address this growing health issue. In this case, the commitment by the district to its policy will lead to the expectation that there will be consistency in the implementation of all related protocols. This, in turn, will lead to a sense of "status quo" regarding related practices and procedures. In other words, these policy procedures will become viewed as "the norm" overtime. The policy should also allow for a process for review, evaluation and revision, when necessary. With this natural and important course of events, it is possible for safe protocols to become standardized and established for students with food allergies.

SUPPLEMENTAL MATERIALS

TEMPLATE FOR
SCHOOL DISTRICT FOOD ALLERGY POLICY

Policy Statement

Compliance with state and federal laws (Section 504 of the Rehabilitation Act of 1973, Americans with Disabilities Act of 1990), related regulations and guidelines

Age appropriate protocols and procedures that address individual needs and enhance a safe learning environment

Commitment to implementation of food allergen management practices which utilize avoidance practices

Physical, social and emotional needs of all students addressed

Individual student and building-based emergency response plans will be in place

Background Information

Allergic Reactions & Anaphylaxis

Causes—Food, Insects, Medications, Latex

Asthma as a risk factor

Epinephrine as the drug of choice

Significance of timely response

Purpose and Goal

Education of staff and community—mandatory

Prevention through risk reduction procedures

Emergency Response, including for previously undiagnosed individuals

Identification of students at risk

Individual Healthcare Plans (IHP or 504 Plan, with emergency treatment plan)

Equal access for all students with an LTA to all educational opportunities

Multidisciplinary approach

Communication of policy content and procedures

Policy review, evaluation and revision

Policy Procedures

Responsibility of School Administrative Personnel

Responsibility of School Principal

Responsibility of School Nurse

Responsibility of Teachers

Responsibility of Food Service Director

Responsibility of Custodial Staff

Responsibility of School Transportation Personnel

Responsibility of Before/After School Personnel

Responsibility of Parents

Responsibility of Students

REFERENCES BY NAME

Annotated as footnotes or within the document

APPENDIX

Support Documents

GLOSSARY OF TERMINOLOGY

RECOMMENDED STANDARDS FOR LIFE THREATENING ALLERGY (LTA) DISTRICT POLICY

Policy Statement

- Policy states the district will strive to make its best effort to address the safety needs of its food-allergic student population, within the least restrictive environment possible.

- Policy language must present the fundamental premise that avoidance practices are the key to successful management of food allergies.

- Policy protocols and procedures must be in compliance with state and federal laws which apply to this area, including Section 504 of the Rehabilitation Act of 1973, the Americans with Disabilities Act of 1990, USDA Federal Regulation-7 CFR 15b, and state medication administration regulations.

- Policy language will promote collaboration between school administration, staff and parents.

- Policy language will state intent of district to provide safe access to all aspects of the student's curriculum and extra-curricular activities.

Background Information

- 6%-8% of children are currently affected by food allergies, which is an increase of over 95% over the past ten years.

- The school setting is known to be a high risk environment for students with food allergies.

- Every food-allergic reaction has the potential to develop into an anaphylactic, life-threatening reaction.

- Students diagnosed with both asthma and food allergies are at a higher risk for anaphylaxis and for more severe anaphylaxis.

Purpose and Goal

- Procedures must be in place to:

  o Identify students who are at risk for anaphylaxis

  o Develop healthcare plans which meet the individual needs of each of these students

- Policy language must reference 504 Plans as a viable means of managing food allergies for those students who meet the required qualifications.

- Policy procedures must be in place which allow for a Section 504 Plan evaluation/eligibility meeting to be conducted by a core building review team when a student with life-threatening food allergies has been identified and/or has requested protection under Section 504. This team should include at a minimum, the school nurse, the building principal and the parents.

- Policy procedures must provide for all identified students to have:

  o Either an Individual Healthcare Plan (IHP) or a Section 504 Plan, and

  o An Emergency Treatment Plan

- Both Plans should be agreed upon by the parent, school nurse and the child's physician, and be in place prior to the first day of school.

- Policy language should clearly define staff's role and responsibilities in the implementation of procedures stated within the policy.

- Policy procedures should be age appropriate and meet the needs of each individual student. Individual accommodations may shift as the student advances through the grades.

- Policy language should allow for regular evaluation of protocols and procedures stated within the policy.

- Policy should clearly state that the school district adopts "zero tolerance" for harassment of students with food allergies.

Responsibility of School Administrative Personnel

- Establish system-wide plan to address life-threatening food allergies.

- School administrators must be familiar with all state and federal laws which protect the rights of students with life-threatening food allergies.

- Procedures established for training of all staff, including auxiliary staff, on food allergies, anaphylaxis and EpiPen® administration, held annually in each school.

- Establish protocols for before/after school-sponsored events.

- Establish protocols for school bus transportation to allow for the safe travel of students with food allergies.

- Provide for review and revision of policy and procedures as needed, but at a minimum of every two years.

Responsibility of School Principal

- Assign food-allergic students to EpiPen® trained teacher.

- Letter sent to all parents in classroom with a food-allergic student. Language used states "life-threatening allergy(s)", where medically indicated, and procedures to be implemented.

- Work with school nurse to insure training of staff regarding food allergies, anaphylaxis, EpiPen® administration and to build food allergy management and emergency response protocols.

- Establish plan for substitute teachers in classrooms with food-allergic students.

- Establish safe protocols in the cafeteria, including arrangements for an allergen-free table(s) to be made available in the cafeteria, with a clear plan for safe cleaning and storage.

- Procedures must be in place to insure that there is no isolation of the food-allergic student in the cafeteria.

- Establish appropriate cleaning procedures throughout the building.

- Arrange for communication devices for staff use (e.g. walkie-talkie, cell phone) when traveling throughout the building, outdoors on school grounds and while on field trips.

- Procedures must be in place to allow for school-wide communication several times per year to increase awareness of food allergy issues and procedures.

- Procedures must allow for a mock emergency drill to be performed by staff annually when no students are present.

- Procedures in place to post signs where appropriate.

- Procedures in place to allow for safe participation of LTA students in school-sponsored, before/after school events.

- Support staff in all LTA programs and procedures.

Responsibility of School Nurse

- EpiPen® Administration Policy in compliance with state and federal regulations.

- Standing orders secured for epinephrine in both doses.

- Epinephrine and other lifesaving medicines must be stored safely in the Nurse's Office and never kept in a locked cabinet during the school day.

- Provisions for additional EpiPen®s to be located wherever a student is at most risk, when medically indicated as necessary. Consideration should be given for an EpiPen® to be kept in the classroom, which would travel with an adult staff member (or the student when appropriate) as the student moves throughout the building and grounds.

- Training of staff in EpiPen® administration, food allergies and anaphylaxis.

- Identify food-allergic students and initiate meeting with each food-allergic student and his/her parents to develop student's healthcare plans.

- Oversee implementation of student's healthcare plans and support staff in their efforts.

- Procedures in place for field trips that allow for:

  o a school nurse to be present on all field trips attended by a student with severe food allergies, or, when this is not possible,

  o a staff member trained in EpiPen® administration to be present on the field trip.

- Procedures in place to make medical information readily available for a substitute nurse in the event that the school nurse is absent.

- Procedures in place to access 911 for medical assistance and transportation of the individual to the hospital, should an EpiPen® be administered.

Responsibility of Teachers

- Receive EpiPen® training and be willing to administer EpiPen® if required.

- Procedures in place to address avoidance of food allergens in curriculum, including in all "specialist" teacher classrooms, such as art, computer, library, music, gym.

- Procedures in place for safe foods used in snack programs and celebrations, especially at the elementary level, in those classrooms with students identified as having life-threatening food allergies.

- Procedures in place to address hand washing/surface washing practices in the classroom.

- Procedures in place for the food-allergic student's safe participation in the cafeteria, without being isolated.

- Procedures in place for field trips which: 1.) allow for the safe participation of the food-allergic student, 2.) provide advance notice to the school nurse for medical coverage and to the parents to allow for their participation.

- Procedures are implemented which are consistent with accommodations outlined in student's individual healthcare plan (IHP).

- LTA procedures accessible for substitute teacher to follow.

Responsibility of Food Service Director

- Follows USDA regulation 7 CFR 15b, "Accommodations for Students with Special Dietary Needs", and provides for safe food substitutions to be made at no extra cost for students with food allergies who buy lunch, per USDA Child Nutrition Services requirements.

- Procedures must be in place to train food service personnel in safe food preparation and cleaning practices.

- Latex-free gloves used when handling food and utensils.

- Allergen-free table(s) is established as needed.

- Identification of students with life-threatening food allergies is established.

- Consider limiting and/or prohibiting the sale of certain 'high risk" foods.

Responsibility of Custodial Staff

- Cleaning of all surfaces with non-allergenic products, and that include a soap surfactant.

- Dedicated bucket and cloth used for allergen-free table surfaces.

Responsibility of School Transportation Personnel

- Procedures established to identify students with food allergies.

- Procedures established to insure the presence of a working communication device.

- Procedures in place to establish a "no eating" rule.

- Emergency Response Plan is in place to be followed in the event of an allergic reaction and/or anaphylaxis.

- Emergency Treatment Plan and EpiPen® are readily accessible.

Responsibility of Parents

- Documentation provided to school of child's life-threatening food allergies and medical history.

- All life-saving medicines are provided in a timely fashion.

- Works with school nurse to develop child's individual healthcare plan and emergency treatment plan.

- Provides safe foods for their child.

- Medic Alert identification provided for their child (recommended).

Responsibility of Students

- No consumption of food with unsafe or unknown ingredients.

- Notification to an adult if an allergic reaction is suspected.

- Understands their role regarding the EpiPen® (for transportation and administration).

SUPPORT DOCUMENTS RECOMMENDED FOR A SCHOOL DISTRICT POLICY

- "Managing Life Threatening Food Allergies" (Guidelines— Massachusetts Department of Elementary and Secondary Education) www.doe.mass.edu/cnp/allergy.pdf.

- "Individualized Health Care Plans (IHP)" (2008 Position Statement, National Association of School Nurses) www. nasn.org/PolicyAdvocacy/PositionPapersandReports/NASNPositionStatementsFullView/tabid/462/.

- "Accommodating Children with Special Dietary Needs in the School Nutrition Programs" (Guidance—United States Department of Agriculture, Food and Nutrition Service) www.fns.usda.gov/cnd/guidance/special_dietary_needs.pdf.

- "Anaphylaxis In Schools And Other Childcare Settings" (1998 Position Statement, American Academy of Allergy, Asthma, and Immunology) www.aaaai.org/practice-resources/statements-and-parameters.aspx.

- "Food Allergies—Key Points" (Educating For Food Allergies, LLC)

- Individual Healthcare Plan Form (Educating For Food Allergies, LLC)

- "Master Checklist for Individualized Healthcare Plans" (Educating For Food Allergies, LLC)

- Emergency Treatment Plan Forms (Educating For Food Allergies, LLC, Food Allergy & Anaphylaxis Network, Asthma and Allergy Foundation of America)

- "IHP vs. 504 Plan Accommodations" (Educating For Food Allergies, LLC)

- "Food-Free Birthday Celebration Ideas" (Educating For Food Allergies, LLC)

"Energy and persistence conquer all things."

Benjamin Franklin

CHAPTER FOUR

THE LAWS AND HOW THEY RELATE TO FOOD ALLERGIES

There are state and federal laws and regulations which have been constructed to protect the rights and privileges of individuals with disabilities, and that includes students with documented life-threatening food allergies. The three federal laws which are most often referred to when we speak about students with life-threatening food allergies are *Section 504 of the Rehabilitation Act of 1973*, the *Americans with Disabilities Act of 1990,* and the *Individuals with Disabilities Education Act*. The discussion of the laws covered in this chapter is intended to demystify and clarify their language so that we may better understand their meaning. It will also help to highlight the ways in which they may be applied to students diagnosed with a food allergy. In other words, it should become clear that students with food allergies should be able to attend schools safely and receive the same benefits of their educational program as those received by students without disabilities. Schools have a responsibility to provide a safe environment for *all* children while providing the resources and opportunities necessary for them to thrive educationally. It is critical, therefore, that school staff and parents understand which laws relate to students with food allergies and have a clear understanding of how to interpret and apply them appropriately.

"Allergy" Defined as a Disability

A persistent source of confusion which I will address first is the question, "Is a student with a life-threatening food allergy considered to have a disability under the law, and if so, why?" In order to answer this question, it is important to understand that the Office for Civil Rights (OCR), within the United States Department of Education, recognizes *allergy* as a "hidden disability". The OCR defines hidden disabilities as "physical or mental impairments that are not readily apparent to others". A physical or mental impairment is defined as "any physiological disorder or condition . . . affecting one or more body systems". In addition, the physical or mental impairment in question must substantially limit one or more major life activities. A "major life activity" would include such things as seeing, hearing, breathing, eating and learning. We know from earlier discussions in the book that an individual with a food allergy may experience substantially limited breathing during anaphylaxis due to the involvement of the body's respiratory system. The physiological condition of a food allergy may also affect the digestive, skin and cardiovascular body systems. Therefore, a life-threatening food allergy meets the criteria of a qualifying impairment, and as such, meets the definition of a disability as offered by the OCR. Why is this important? Meeting the definition of a disability is significant for an individual with a documented life-threatening food allergy because it means that he or she is protected under both state and federal laws.

DISABILITY AND EDUCATION RIGHTS

Attorneys and other advocates and consultants should facilitate constructive, informed dialogue between parents and school administrators. Whenever possible, the parents should be in the foreground and their relationships with school staff and administrators should be primary. Successful advocates walk away from empowered, informed parents, able to continue forward independently. Resources such as this volume can be an important tool in the parent education and empowerment process.

This degree of success, however, is not always possible; sometimes one party simply cannot hear or acknowledge the other. In my experience, this often leads to the finger-pointing or blame-assigning stage of the parent/school relationship. This relationship is circular and, therefore, potentially endless.

With stakes as high as a life-threatening allergy, finger-pointing is a reckless luxury. If parents come to believe that, despite their best efforts, their child is unsafe in school, they should be helped and encouraged in exploring their enforcement options and the relief available from each. At this point, many parents will want to consult with a disability rights organization or an attorney knowledgeable about disability rights, or education rights, or both.

It is not necessary to exclude consultants whose support and expertise is still desired; rather, the parents should ensure that all team members are able to work cooperatively, that roles are clear and appropriate and that all efforts are guided by the parents' informed decisions.

Ray Wallace, Attorney, Wallace Law Office, PC,
Canton, Massachusetts

Section 504 of the Rehabilitation Act of 1973 (PL 93-112)

Because students who have been diagnosed with a life-threatening food allergy are generally considered to have a disability, they may be eligible for protection under Section 504 of the Rehabilitation Act of 1973. Section 504 is a civil rights law which is enforced by the OCR, within the U.S. Department of Education. This federal law was constructed to protect the rights of individuals with a disability and says specifically that it is meant to: "prohibit discrimination on the basis of disability in education . . . in any program or institution receiving federal funds, and to ensure that students with handicaps or disabilities receive a free appropriate education." This statement, when looked at closely, has several important implications. First, any public entity or program that receives federal funding for any reason must comply with the requirements found under Section 504. Most, if not all, public school systems are recipients of federal monies in the form of financial assistance (known as federal financial assistance, or FFA's), to such things as school lunch programs. When a school district makes arrangements to receive federal money for *any* school-sponsored program, they are, in effect, signing a contract with the government which says they agree not to discriminate against anyone with a disability and uphold the requirements set forth in this law. It should be noted that since most colleges and universities receive some form of federal funding, students with disabilities who attend these institutions are protected under Section 504. It is also important to realize that private schools are also required to comply with the provisions found under Section 504 if they receive federal funding for any reason.

A Free Appropriate Education (FAPE)

Secondly, Section 504 states specifically that individuals with disabilities must receive a "free appropriate education", which is often referred to as "FAPE". Simply put, this means that disabled students must be educated alongside students without disabilities, to the fullest extent possible. In other words, FAPE requirements prohibit assigning disabled students to segregated classes or facilities in elementary, secondary and post-secondary schools. Only when, even with the assistance of auxiliary aids and services, the disabled student is not able to progress educationally, may the student be assigned to a separate class. The word, "appropriate", means that whenever possible, the educational program and related curriculum must accommodate the safe inclusion of ***all*** students, including in such areas as art, music, physical education, lunch, recess, field trips, etc.

Does 504 protection extend to non-academic services and programs offered by the school which take place after school hours? Again, the answer is yes. Students may not be excluded from participating in extracurricular activities sponsored by the school based on their disability alone, including in recreational, sports or club activities and after-school care programs. Complying with the law cannot be based on what is convenient. Schools that have made an agreement with the federal government to receive funding can not simply pick and choose the time of day they will engage in activities which would be considered nondiscriminatory. This means that a school must make arrangements for the student with Section 504 protection to be able to participate safely in the after school activities of the student's choice. Whether this means involvement on a school team sport or attending a school-sponsored dance, it is the responsibility of the school to make appropriate accommodations for that student. This does not always mean that the school nurse must be present at the after school program attended by the student with food allergies. Many schools address this obligation by making arrangements for the student's medicine, such as the EpiPen®, to be readily accessible, in addition to having a properly trained adult staff member on site who would be able to administer the medicine, should the student require treatment for an allergic reaction.

In addition, FAPE requires that inclusion in these programs must be made at no extra cost to the student with the disability or his/her family, regardless of whether aids or special services are required. For students with food allergies, the need for special services might be for an aide to be present during lunch at the elementary school level to insure that children are not sharing food and possible allergens. Similarly, an aide may be utilized on the school bus so that children with life-threatening food allergies may ride safely with their peers. Another example of a special service would be the need for medication, such as epinephrine prescribed by a doctor, to be administered. Schools that have a full-time nurse generally have no problem supplying this service, however, schools with only a part-time nurse, or in some cases with no nurse at all, may experience some difficulties fulfilling this need. Schools in this predicament must still find a way to administer required medications appropriately and within the confines of legal nursing practices and they must do this at no additional cost to the families who require this service. This may be a particular challenge to some school districts given the fact that Section 504 does not offer state or federal funding to assist the district in complying with its implementation. In other words, all costs incurred by the district to meet its obligation under Section 504 are the sole responsibility of the district. The safety of the student is not expendable, however, regardless of whether budget problems exist. Schools have a duty to care for all of their students because it is the right thing to do, and for their students with special needs, because it is also required under the law.

SECTION 504 PLANS

Students with a documented life-threatening food allergy (written documentation from the student's physician which verifies this diagnosis) may qualify for protection under Section 504 of the Rehabilitation Act of 1973 in the form of a 504 Plan. A 504 Plan, which is considered a legal document, is a product of the provisions found in Section 504. It establishes formal healthcare accommodations for students with special health care needs so that they may enjoy the benefits of their educational program.

Formal Request and Evaluation Meeting

Who may request that a student be considered for a 504 Plan? The answer is anyone familiar with the child and his/her needs. This could be the child's teacher, the school nurse, and the principal, or the child's parents, for example. It is, in fact, the obligation and responsibility of any school which receives federal funding to, on an annual basis, identify any individual who may be eligible for protection under Section 504. Each school building within the district should have a staff member assigned Section 504 compliance responsibilities. Therefore, whoever makes the request that a student be considered for Section 504 protection should do so in writing and direct it to the attention of either 1.) the head of school (principal, headmaster or director, for example) with a request that the letter be directed to the school employee who has been assigned Section 504 compliance responsibilities, or 2.) the school district's administrator responsible for students with special needs and Section 504 compliance (often called the Director of Student Services or the Director of Special Education).

Once a formal request has been made, the law requires that a formal evaluation meeting will be held to determine the student's eligibility for Section 504 protection, and that the parents will be notified of the impending evaluation meeting. The law also requires that parents are informed of their rights regarding this process and the name of the person to contact should they have questions or concerns. In addition, there must be a formal process for grievance issues and for the resolution of complaints. Therefore, a school district will have a "Parent's Rights Brochure", or some similarly named document, which will outline the required information. Lastly, Section 504 requires that parents are notified of the meeting's outcome.

Parents are not required to be at this evaluation meeting, but not only is it the appropriate thing to do, it usually results in a better outcome for the student because the parents are able to share insights and information about their child's health issue. Therefore, having the parents of the child in question attend this meeting is considered to be the best practice. The OCR, in their informational pamphlet, "The Civil Rights of Students with Hidden Disabilities Under Section 504 of the Rehabilitation Act of 1973" states that it is the responsibility of any school which receives federal funds to "establish procedural safeguards to enable parents and guardians to participate meaningfully in decisions regarding the evaluation and placement of their children".

If a child is determined to meet the qualifications for a 504 Plan, a planning team will be assembled by the staff person responsible for Section 504 compliance. The goal of this meeting is to develop accommodations meant to meet the student's individual health needs. The child's parents are not required to be members of the 504 planning team, nor is their signature indicating approval of the 504 Plan required under this law, however, once again, it is considered to be the best practice. Members of a 504 planning team typically include the school nurse, the school principal, the classroom teacher, a staff member assigned the responsibility of overseeing Section 504 issues (if this is not one of the individuals already mentioned here), and the child's parents, however the composition of this team will vary from school to school.

An "accommodation" listed on the child's 504 Plan refers to any procedure that will be followed which enable the child to enjoy the same benefits and opportunities as the child's nondisabled counterparts. Words like, "We haven't ever done anything like that before", which may be given as a reason not to make a particular accommodation, are unacceptable. Disability laws require that decisions regarding the nature of an accommodation be based on the *individual* needs of the student and not on what is either easiest or has been done before. Therefore, specific strategies for each individual student's educational program must be made to help enhance *that* student's safety and full participation in activities while at school. (refer to Chapter 3 for more information on Section 504 Plans)

SECTION 504 PLANS: A PARENT'S PERSPECTIVE

Just before my son entered kindergarten in the public schools, I had a long talk with the principal, nurse and classroom teacher about his life-threatening food allergies and what the protocol would be if he were to have a reaction. I felt confident that everyone understood the seriousness of the issue and their respective roles in keeping him safe. At Christmas-time, the teacher decided without my knowledge to have the children make gingerbread houses with egg-based frosting at the end of the day. I went to pick up my son, and he was covered from head to toe in hives, in the midst of an anaphylactic reaction. No one in the school had noticed, so I gave him an EpiPen® and took him to the emergency room. When I confronted the teacher the next day, she tried to blame my son, saying that he did not tell her he was having a reaction, so she didn't notice, but she did tell him he could "lick his fingers clean" instead of using the sink. In addition to the physical harm of the reaction, he suffered emotionally and did not want to enter the cafeteria where the reaction had happened. Because I never wanted him to suffer a reaction at school again, I immediately made arrangements for my son to have a written 504 Plan, which included among other things his wearing his EpiPen® on his belt, that I have documentation that all the teachers were properly EpiPen® trained, and that the children wash their hands before the start of the day and after lunch. Despite all we had been through, the teacher initially refused to comply with the plan, stating that it was "too difficult to get 20 kindergarteners to wash their hands." I was forced to file a complaint with the compliance department of the Massachusetts Department of Education. After some legal wrangling, the teacher relented and agreed to all the provisions in the 504 Plan. I learned my lesson not to assume that everyone in the school understands how to handle food allergies properly. I now insist on a written, legally-enforceable 504 Plan at the beginning of

> each school year so it is clear what needs to be done to keep him safe. My son has not had another reaction in school. The administration now understands the seriousness of the issue, and they understand how serious I am about keeping him safe.
>
> Laurel Francouer, Parent
> Woburn, Massachusetts

Liability Waivers

During the process of planning appropriate accommodations for a child with food allergies, it appears that some school officials believe it is appropriate to ask the parents to sign a liability waiver stating that the school would not be held legally accountable should their child be harmed while under the school's care. In some instances, school administrators have stated that unless the parents sign this waiver, staff will not administer medicines, regardless of whether those medicines are needed. This is not appropriate. An administrator may not arbitrarily decide whether staff will administer a student's medicine. In fact, the OCR has ruled that if a child needs medicine in order to attend school, then the school is obligated to administer it. The OCR has also ruled that if a school refuses to administer medicine without a signed waiver, it is in violation of Section 504. School staff have the basic duty and responsibility to address the safety of all of their students, and to make reasonable efforts to do so.

Family Educational Rights and Privacy Act (FERPA)

Once a 504 Plan has been developed for a student, it is the expectation that accommodations in the plan, which are meant to address the student's safety at school, will be implemented by designated school staff, such as the school nurse and the student's teachers. Some parents and school administrators are concerned about whether the student's healthcare plan, which often includes the student's picture and other indentifying information, should be shared with school staff other than the school nurse. The Family Educational Rights and Privacy Act (FERPA), is a federal law which requires any public or private school which receives federal funding to protect the privacy of student education records. Under FERPA, a student's health record may be shared with teachers and other appropriate school officials in connection with an emergency, when such knowledge is essential to protect the health and well-being of the student. Therefore, it is reasonable that a student's 504 Plan (or an Individual Healthcare Plan) and Emergency Treatment Plan should be shared with school staff for which this information is necessary, in order to help them protect the welfare of the student. This doesn't mean that students' health plans should be posted in public areas for everyone to see. Rather, they should be kept in areas where only those who have a legitimate need to know may access this information. (For more information about FERPA, contact: Family Policy Compliance Office, U.S. Department of Education, 400 Maryland Avenue, S.W., Washington, D.C. 20202-8520, or go to: www.ed.gov/policy/gen/guid/fpco/index.html)

Safe Inclusion may Require Modifications to the Curriculum

The purpose of a 504 Plan is to allow the student to be able to safely take advantage of all aspects of the educational program being presented. Classroom materials that would put the student with food allergies at risk should not be used. Teachers will need to make modifications to their academic or extra-curricular programs, when this is the case, in order to follow the student's 504 Plan and meet the special needs of the student. Telling the child not to come to school on a certain day because of a project which is planned that contains materials to which the student is allergic, or sending the student to another room while a lesson is being taught, are not options. In other words, the teacher must find a way to safely include the student in the classroom curriculum being presented.

Author's Note

A few years ago I was made aware of a high school student with a documented, severe nut allergy who was enrolled in a home economics cooking class. Her teacher insisted on using nuts as part of the ingredients in various recipes. Although the student informed the teacher that cooking nuts would aerosolize the proteins into the air, and consequently put her at risk for an allergic reaction and possible anaphylaxis, the teacher refused to substitute the allergen for another ingredient. Instead, she suggested that the student simply go to the library during classes when the nuts were being baked. This action taken by the teacher is a violation of civil rights law and is discriminatory because it segregated the student from her peers and denied her access to the same benefits of the educational program being received by her nondisabled classmates. A simple solution and an appropriate response to this situation would have been for the teacher to either remove the foods to which the student was allergic and replace them with alternative ingredients, or to have used a different recipe which didn't include any of the student's allergies. *In the end, the student's parents asked for and went through the process for a 504 Plan for their child which delineated specific risk reduction practices the teacher needed to follow in order to maintain the student's health. Nuts were no longer used during the student's class time.*

More information on 504 Plans may be found in Chapter 3. The Office for Civil Rights, within the U.S. Department of Education, holds its main office in Washington, D.C., but maintains twelve regional offices throughout the United States. OCR headquarters may be contacted at the: U.S. Department of Education, Office for Civil Rights, 400 Maryland Avenue, S.W., Washington, DC 20202-1100. They can be reached by phone at: (800)421-3481.

Individuals with Disabilities Education Act (IDEA)

The Individuals with Disabilities Education Act, commonly referred to as IDEA, is administered by the Office of Special Education & Rehabilitative Services, within the U.S. Department of Education. It is a federal, special education law and was written to ensure that children with disabilities receive the services necessary " . . . to allow them to benefit from their educational program." *Simply stated, this law is intended to protect the rights of children who have a disability that hinders their ability to learn and therefore can not make reasonable progress at school.* This Act requires that special education and related services be provided.

The IDEA has thirteen formal designations for disabilities, whereas the definition for a disability under Section 504 is much broader (refer to "Section 504 vs. IDEA" at the end of the chapter under "Supplemental Materials" for a list of these disabilities). A student determined to have one of these thirteen disabilities is entitled to receive a free and appropriate education, or FAPE as it was referenced earlier in this chapter. Under IDEA, federal funding is given to states to assist them with their costs in providing any educational aid or service extended to a student, and these services must be made at no extra cost to the family.

If a student has a handicap that affects their ability to learn, they will likely need special assistance in order to progress satisfactorily with their academic program. When it is determined that a student needs special education teacher instructional services, then a written plan called an *"Individualized Education Plan"*, or *"IEP"*, must be developed to enable that child to meet their educational goals. Parents must receive *written* notice if their child is being evaluated for an IEP. In addition, they are required to be part of the planning team for their child's written educational plan, and their signature signifying acceptance of the plan is required.

It is possible that a student with food allergies may also have a disability which affects his/her learning. An example of this would be a child with a food allergy who also has asthma so acute that the child misses school to the extent that he or she has difficulty keeping up with the curriculum. In this scenario, the child would require protection under the IDEA, and would receive an IEP, rather than a 504 Plan. The IEP in this case would address both the student's learning disability as covered under IDEA, and the student's health needs, as provided for under Section 504 (in this case, a 504 Plan would be an attachment to the student's IEP). If, on the other hand, a student with life-threatening food allergies has asthma which is well-controlled and is therefore able to handle the classroom curriculum presented, the student would receive protection under Section 504.

For more information about the IDEA, please contact the: Office of Special Education and Rehabilitative Services, U.S. Department of Education, 400 Maryland Avenue, S.W., Washington, D.C., 20202-7100. This office may be reached by phone at (202)245-7408.

Americans with Disabilities Act of 1990

The Americans with Disabilities Act of 1990, most often referred to as the ADA, is a federal civil rights law enforced by the U.S. Department of Justice. This law was constructed with the clear purpose of eliminating discrimination against anyone with a disability. Its language provides mandates which are intended to set standards to insure that people with disabilities have opportunities equal to people without disabilities. The law clearly states that " . . . no individual shall be discriminated against on the basis of disability in the full and equal enjoyment of the goods, services, facilities, privileges, advantages . . . of any place of public accommodation . . ."

Title II and Title III

There are two sections called "Titles" within the ADA which may be applied to students with life-threatening food allergies: **Title II and Title III.** The requirements of Title II are similar to those found in Section 504. They state that no qualified person with a disability may be " . . . excluded from participation in or be denied the benefits of services, programs or activities of a public entity . . .". A "public entity" may be defined as any state or local government or its agency. Title II, therefore, refers to individuals with disabilities in state and local government agencies and programs and says that these programs must be readily accessible to them. A public school is an example of a government agency. This means that public schools, under the ADA, must provide educational opportunities and activities which allow their disabled students to participate safely and receive the same benefits of their education as their nondisabled students. Similarly, public childcare centers which are run by state or local government agencies, such as Head Start and after school programs, must also comply with Title II of the ADA.

Title III of the ADA extends these same rights to individuals with disabilities in places of public accommodation *regardless of whether they receive federal funds.* This makes the requirements presented by the ADA broader than those found under Section 504. Included within the definition of places of public accommodation by a private entity are: "a nursery, elementary, secondary, undergraduate or postgraduate private school". In other words, students with diagnosed life-threatening food allergies who attend private schools, preschools and daycare centers are entitled to the same educational benefits as the rest of their classmates. Like their public counterparts, these private institutions must be prepared to appropriately handle the needs of their students with food allergies, such as administering epinephrine to a student experiencing anaphylaxis. If a school does not have a nurse, it is the obligation of the school to train someone in the proper technique of administering medically required medicines and assign that person with that responsibility.

Mediation Program

In 1994, the ADA established a Mediation Program as a means of resolving disputes by utilizing informal procedures. Participation in mediation is voluntary and requires that there be an impartial third party assigned whose role it is to make sure that the process is fair to both parties involved in the conflict. If mediation efforts prove unsuccessful in soliciting a resolution, legal recourse may be pursued under the ADA. (refer to section in this chapter on Formal Grievance Procedures)

For more information about the ADA, please contact the: U.S. Department of Justice, Civil Rights Division, Disability Rights Section – NYA, 950 Pennsylvania Avenue, N.W., Washington, D.C., 20530. The toll free ADA Information Line is: (800) 514-0301.

FORMAL GRIEVANCE PROCEDURES

Most school administrators today understand that children with food allergies have special health needs and require assistance in some way to allow them to attend school safely and enjoy the same educational opportunities as their peers. Unfortunately, however, some school personnel do not seem to recognize or understand this need. This may be due, in part, to a general misunderstanding of civil rights laws and the school's obligations under these laws. As a result, school practices may exist which pose a barrier to the safe inclusion of all students. When a child becomes the victim of an unsafe environment, less than equal educational opportunities, or is being excluded, stigmatized or harassed, it is important to know that parents have the right to pursue a resolution to this treatment by utilizing the due process procedures provided by the civil rights laws previously discussed. There is rarely just one place to turn for a violation of a child's right to an appropriate accommodation. There are federal and state resources for solving disputes, often with overlapping authority. If a formal complaint to a federal or state agency or court becomes necessary, it is wise to consult an attorney knowledgeable in civil rights laws, if possible, before deciding which claim to bring and to which forum.

FEDERAL GRIEVANCE PROCEDURES

For Section 504 and the ADA, Title II

There may be circumstances when a student with disabilities, or the student's family, believe that the student has been discriminated against. The Office for Civil Rights, within the U.S. Department of Education, enforces federal civil rights laws. Specifically, they enforce the anti-discrimination requirements of Section 504 of the Rehabilitation Act of 1973 and Title II of the Americans with Disabilities Act of 1990. Section 504 requires that schools have formal grievance procedures for occasions such as this. This means that the district must designate a staff member as the compliance officer to oversee this process. If attempts at resolving the problem do not work at the local level, then a formal complaint may be filed with the OCR by the child, the parent, or some other person acting on behalf of that child. It is important to understand that a complaint needs to be filed within 180 days from the date of the last act of the alleged discrimination.

Reasons to file a formal complaint might be the refusal by the school district to consider a child with documented life-threatening food allergies for a 504 Plan, having accommodations which are considered to be insufficient, the belief that accommodations within a 504 Plan are not being implemented in good faith or when the child with food allergies is being bullied, which would be considered harassment. In addition, a public entity such as a school that receives federal funding, may not refuse entry of a student with a disability to their program, based simply on the fact that the child has a disability. This would be considered discriminatory and in violation of civil rights law, and would therefore be just cause for filing a grievance with the OCR.

There are four ways to communicate with the OCR:

Mail: Office for Civil Rights, US Dept. of Education, 400
            Maryland Ave., S.W., Washington, DC 20202-1100

Fax: (202) 245-6840,

Email: ocr@ed.gov,

Online: www.ed.gov/about/offices/list/ocr/complaintintro.html
            where an electronic complaint form may be accessed.

The OCR's regional office contact information may be found on the website listed above. The best way to file a complaint, however, is to send the OCR an email. Regardless of which method of communication you prefer, the following information should be included: 1.) the name and address of the person making the complaint (including a telephone number is helpful), 2.) a description of the person who is the subject of the alleged discrimination (the person's name is not required), 3.) a detailed description of the circumstances of the event(s), and 4.) the name and address of the organization believed to have committed the discriminatory act(s).

Once a complaint has been filed, the OCR will investigate the circumstances of the charges. Whenever possible, the OCR tries first to resolve the problem through discussion and negotiation with both the school and the family. If these efforts do not prove to be productive, however, the school district must provide an impartial hearing in order to resolve the issue(s) in question. The law also requires that parents are given the opportunity to be involved at the hearing and have their voices heard. If an organization is found to be responsible for discrimination against an individual based on their disability, then the OCR may decide to suspend federal financial assistance to that organization. An example of this would be the monies provided from the National School Meal Program given to the school to reduce costs for its school lunch program. In some cases, the OCR may refer the case to the Department of Justice for further review and action.

For the ADA, Title III

Complaints of civil rights violations under Title III of the Americans with Disabilities Act may be filed with the Civil Rights Division within the U.S. Department of Justice. All complaints should be put in writing and sent to the following address: U.S. Department of Justice, Civil Rights Division, Disability Rights Section—NYA, 950 Pennsylvania Avenue, N.W., Washington, D.C., 20530. The letter of complaint should include the following information: 1.) the name, address and phone number of the person being discriminated against, 2.) the name of the business or organization being accused of discrimination, and 3.) a description of the discriminatory act(s), including dates and the name(s) of the individuals involved. Once the Civil Rights Division receives this letter, it will consider all aspects of the complaint and decide which course of action it wishes to take. It is possible for the Division to request additional information, and in some cases, it may decide to pursue legal action, such as a lawsuit.

Example of a case heard by the U.S. Department of Justice

Failure to comply with the ADA can be very serious and may result in civil and criminal penalties. A court case involving the U.S. Department of Justice and La Petite Academy, Inc., which reached a settlement agreement in 1997, demonstrates this point. This case is of particular significance because it addresses accommodations for students with food allergies. The courts found that La Petite Academy was not providing reasonable modifications to their childcare program for its children with disabilities. As a result, La Petite Academy, Inc. was ordered to pay monetary damages in the amount of $55,000 to five children, three of whom have food allergies, as a result of the school's discriminatory actions. Furthermore, the agreement requires this national childcare provider to keep a child's prescribed epinephrine on hand, and to administer an EpiPen® auto-injector, if authorized by the parent and physician, to any student who is having a life-threatening allergic reaction to a food or bee sting. (This settlement agreement may be found at www.usdoj.gov/crt/ada/lapetite.htm.)

STATE GRIEVANCE PROCEDURES

If a state is a recipient of IDEA funding, as is currently the case for all states, it is required to have a "fair hearing" process in place in order to address disputes when they arise. For some states, Rhode Island, for example, this grievance process begins with a hearing officer who represents the local school district. If an adverse decision is made, the parties involved may appeal the decision to a state hearing officer. In other states, however, the grievance process begins with a state-run office designed to handle issues regarding discrimination based on disability. An example of such an office is the **Bureau of Special Education Appeals (BSEA)** which was formed by the Massachusetts Department of Education in order to facilitate procedures for the due process rights of students, parents and public and private schools. The BSEA operates independently from the MA Department of Education. Its purpose is to resolve complaints or differences of opinion between schools and families over the educational programs of special needs students, when they can't be resolved at the local school district level. It has the authority to resolve these conflicts under both state law and federal law (Section 504 and IDEA, for example).

Complaints brought to the MA BSEA may be made by the parents of the student in question, as may a representative of the school district, and either party may be accompanied by an attorney or advocate to the hearing. The Bureau schedules a hearing date thirty-five days after the receipt of a hearing request and holds impartial hearings that follow

hearing rules conducted under the Formal Standard
Rules of Practice and Procedure, 801 CMR 1.01 *et se(*
follows a prescribed format and decisions made by the I
who is an attorney, are based on facts and evidence p..._
hearings. These state-run offices are a great resource to parents and
schools. In many instances they are able to expedite the due process
system and render a decision more quickly than at the federal level.

It is important to understand that federal rules govern the scheduling
and conduct of administrative hearings. In addition, state hearing
officers' decisions can be reviewed by state or federal courts. In
order to determine the manner in which your state conducts its "fair
hearing" process, contact the Superintendent at your local school
district, or your State Department of Education.

Massachusetts Bureau of Special Education Appeals, Case #03-3629

This actual case is of particular interest to the issue of
reasonable accommodations for students with life-threatening
food allergies. It involved a seven year old student who has
asthma, a documented life-threatening allergy to peanuts/nuts, a
history of mild to severe allergic reactions and anaphylaxis. The
student's family requested that there be a ban on peanuts/nuts in
the classroom and that the responsibility for the student's safety
rest primarily with adult staff. The school (a Charter school)
maintained that a ban on peanuts/nuts in the classroom was too
difficult to enforce and therefore placed an undue burden on
staff, and that such a ban would raise a false sense of security.
The school had assigned the student to eat in an allergy-free
"zone" with one other child, and placed the responsibility of
monitoring the medical condition of the student directly on the
student. At the conclusion of the hearing, the Hearing Officer
made the following decisions:

1.) An allergen-free "zone" is insufficient to protect the safety of the student due to the history of a near-fatal reaction. A decision was made to make the room allergen-free.

(When considering an accommodation, the BSEA looks at the impact of the modification on the rights of the other students in the class, in regards to their education and how the modification would affect their education. In this case, they found no evidence that a peanut/nut ban would affect the integrity of the educational program.)

2.) The practice of having the allergic student sit with only one other student was found to be "discriminatory".

3.) Adults must bear the responsibility to keep the allergic student safe. (This meant that adult staff would be responsible to carry the student's EpiPen® and treatment plan to all specialists and functions held outside the classroom.)

4.) The student must have access to *all* classroom activities.

5.) The letter sent to classmates' parents must use language that states specifically that the student has a "life-threatening allergy".

ASTHMATIC SCHOOL CHILDREN'S TREATMENT AND HEALTH MANAGEMENT ACT OF 2004

This federal law (Public Law 108-377) which was signed into effect by President Bush in October, 2004, is codified at 42 U.S.C. § 2809. It is intended to help school children who have asthma or allergic health conditions have the ability to access their medicine when they need it. Students may carry and self-administer medicine for asthma or anaphylaxis under certain conditions, if 1.) the medicine is prescribed by a health care practitioner for use during school hours, 2.) the student is instructed on the proper use of the medicine, and demonstrates the skills necessary to correctly administer it, and 3.)

the student's parent or guardian submits signed permission for their child to carry and self-administer the medicine.

The impact of this law in states that have adopted it is significant in two important ways. First, it provides an effective means for students who meet the above criteria to quickly access their inhaler or EpiPen®. This will greatly reduce the amount of time between the first signs of a medical emergency and treatment. Research has demonstrated that epinephrine, when administered promptly, increases the effectiveness of the medication, which tends to result in a more positive outcome. Second, under this law and in accordance with its requirements, any state which allows students to carry and self-administer their asthma or anaphylaxis medicine will receive preference by the federal government for asthma-related grants. This particular feature of the law may serve as a catalyst for states to develop policies allowing their students to carry life-saving medicines at school.

USDA FEDERAL REGULATION 7 CFR 15b

Students with diagnosed, life-threatening food allergies who plan to buy lunch provided by the school, have the right to eat foods that do not contain any ingredients to which they are allergic. The U.S. Department of Agriculture, or USDA, has non-discrimination regulations under 7 CFR 15b which requires that safe food substitutions must be made for students whose physicians provide documentation that their handicap restricts their diet, when the school is a participant in the National School Lunch or Breakfast Programs. Typically, all public schools and many private schools participate in these programs and receive federal financial assistance (FFA) to help subsidize the cost of the meals they serve.

In order to assist students with food restrictions, including those with food allergies, to eat safely, and also to be in compliance with all relevant laws and regulations, the USDA, Food and Nutrition

Service (sometimes referred to as the FNS), published a handbook titled, "Accommodating Children with Special Dietary Needs in the School Nutrition Programs", which gives guidance to school food service staff on this issue. It is important to note that in this publication, the definition of "disability", as covered under Section 504, includes "food anaphylaxis" as a physical or mental impairment, and specifically lists "eating" as a major life activity. The inclusion of this definition is particularly helpful to families of children with life-threatening food allergies, because it helps to erase questions which sometimes persist as to whether food allergy may be considered a disability under the law.

Because schools have the responsibility to provide safe meals to a student with a documented, life-threatening food allergy, food service staff will need to check food labels for specific ingredients, including evidence of trace amounts of the allergen in question. Ingredient labels should be kept on file by food service staff as a part of their production records, which also includes such things as recipes and products used. By following these procedures, it becomes easier to check the ingredients in products which have been used for meals, should a child have an allergic reaction. There may be occasions when more information is needed, and in these cases, food service will need to contact the manufacturer directly.

Specific instructions for food service staff can be found in Appendix A of the USDA handbook. Here, the FNS Instruction 783-2, Revision 2, *Meal Substitutions for Medical or Other Special Dietary Reasons*, presents the policy regarding meal substitutions for individuals who are considered to have a disability. When a family requests information on foods used by the school cafeteria, and the need for food substitutions to be made, there are certain procedures which need to be followed by both the family and the school.

<u>Responsibility of the Cafeteria, under USDA Regulations:</u>

1. Staff is required to prepare safe meals of equivalent quality if requested by the family of the food-allergic student

2. This special meal must be provided at <u>no extra cost to the family</u>

<u>Responsibility of the Family, under USDA Regulations:</u>

Parents need to submit signed documentation from their licensed physician to the school nurse which explains:

1. The disability and why it restricts the diet (*e.g.,* life-threatening food allergy)

2. The major life activity affected (*e.g.,* caring for one's self, breathing, eating)

3. The food or foods to be omitted <u>and</u>

4. The foods to be used as substitutions

Food substitutions, in general, can be made relatively easily, and with very little, if any, cost to the school. Good communication between the family and cafeteria staff, including documentation clearly stating which foods need to be avoided and which foods may be used as substitutions, will allow food-allergic students to eat safely at school. This should be viewed as a collaborative effort. Families should meet with school food service staff well in advance, in order for the school to have sufficient time to adequately meet the special needs of their child with food allergies.

...rmation on ways to keep students with food allergies ...afeteria, contact the Child and Nutrition Program ...r State Department of Education. More information ...ded procedures in the cafeteria may be found in Chapter 3.)

Author's Note

I am constantly frustrated by persistent reports of schools that choose to have a food-allergic student eat alone at an allergen-free table in the cafeteria. In other instances, there are schools which have the student with a food allergy leave their friends in the cafeteria and report to the nurse's office to eat his/her lunch there. Either of these instances is discriminatory because they segregate and isolate the student with a food allergy, and in so doing, deny food-allergic children from having the opportunity to interact and engage socially with the rest of their peers during lunch. *Many schools provide an "allergen-free" table in the cafeteria during lunch where children with food allergies may choose to sit for safety reasons. It is important that arrangements be made for other children with "safe" lunches to also sit at this table. Chapter 3 explores, in detail, easy and effective ways to make this happen.*

STATE REGULATIONS OF MEDICINE ADMINISTRATION

Nursing Practices

Each state in the U. S. develops its own rules and regulations by which each nurse in that state must abide. The rules will determine what a nurse may and may not do within their practice, and will include specific rules regarding such things as medication administration. Policies regarding when and how a nurse may delegate the responsibility of administering prescription medications to an individual without a nursing license, are generally included. It is important to note that in some states, this particular responsibility may not be delegated at all.

State Departments of Public Health

Each state in the U.S. has some form of a **Public Health Department** which may dictate the manner in which school nurses may administer medicine. The policies within these regulations vary from state to state. For example, some states have regulations which do not provide for the delegation of life-saving medications, such as epinephrine. Understanding these rules and how they may affect procedures at school are important for the school nurse, school administrators, and parents of children with life-threatening food allergies who may require epinephrine to be administered during the school day. The following information includes examples of state laws regarding epinephrine administration at school.

Massachusetts Department of Public Health

In Massachusetts, the Department of Public Health (DPH) has a regulation, 105 CMR 210.000, which provides standards for maintaining the safe and proper administration of physician-prescribed medications at the elementary and secondary grade levels, for both public and private schools. The policies within this regulation permit a school nurse to delegate the responsibility for administering prescription medications, including epinephrine by auto-injector in a life-threatening situation, to school personnel who don't have a nursing license when a school nurse is not available. Certain criteria must be met when EpiPen® administration is to be delegated. The regulation dictates that this may only happen when the person designated by the nurse has been properly trained (the Massachusetts DPH has a specific curriculum intended for this training), and is supervised by the school nurse. In addition, the school district must fill out an application to register with the Massachusetts DPH for this purpose.

This regulation, which was amended in the fall of 2003, now has specific language which requires that whenever a school district intends to permit the administration of epinephrine by auto-injector by unlicensed school personnel, the district must also implement "a plan for comprehensive risk reduction for the student, including preventing exposure to specific allergens". In other words, in order for the nurse to be able to delegate the administration of epinephrine to an unlicensed staff member, the school *must* develop a thorough plan to manage the student's allergies, including implementing strategies to avoid the offending allergens.

Maine Public Law 2003, Chapter 531

In 2004, the Maine legislature approved Public Law 2003, chapter 531, referred to as, *An Act To Authorize Certain School Children to Carry Emergency Medication on Their Person.* This law, intended for public and private schools, requires that local policy be developed and adopted which allows students to carry epinephrine auto-injectors and/or asthma inhalers, and to self-administer them, if necessary. Schools must receive written authorization from the student's parent or guardian and the student's primary health care provider indicating their approval for this procedure, including verification that the student is capable of carrying and using the epinephrine device and/or inhaler. The school nurse is also responsible for determining the student's skill and ability to properly use the epinephrine auto-injector or asthma inhaler before permission is granted to do so.

New Hampshire Chapter 50, Section 2-4 and Section 6-8

House Bill 92, titled *Use of Epinephrine Auto-Injectors by Pupils and Campers with Severe Allergies*, was enacted into law as Chapter 50 in 2003 by the New Hampshire Legislature. Section 2-4 of this Act permits epinephrine auto-injectors to be carried and self-administered by a student with severe allergies, as long as the student has written approval from a physician, including related information such as verification that the student has the appropriate skills to safely carry and use this device. Students under the age of eighteen must also have written permission from their parents or guardians. Copies of written approval must be in the possession of the school nurse or school principal. Permission to carry and use an epinephrine auto-injector applies to the school day, including any school-sponsored event, activity or program. This law calls for the school nurse, or school principal if there is not a nurse, to maintain at least one epinephrine auto-injector (provided by the student), in the nurse's office or other accessible location.

Section 6-8 of this Act pertains to epinephrine auto-injectors which are carried and used at recreation camps. The conditions which must be met in order for a child to carry and potentially self-administer this medication at camp are similar to those found in Section 2-4. It is important to recognize that in the State of New Hampshire, by the requirements of this law, **a second epinephrine auto-injector *must* be maintained and made available** for students or campers who have been given permission to carry their own epinephrine device.

(Note: As of May, 2012, 48 States, including the District of Columbia, have laws which allow students to carry epinephrine by auto-injector. Check with your own state to determine whether and how epinephrine may be carried and administered at school.)

GOOD SAMARITAN LAWS

Students with food allergies need to have epinephrine, a potentially lifesaving medicine, readily accessible, and someone competent to administer it, should they experience an allergic reaction. School employees may have concerns that they could be held legally accountable, should they administer emergency medicine and something was to go wrong. As a result, most states have a "Good Samaritan" law which protects public school employees who provide emergency medical care to an individual to the best of their ability from civil liability. For example, in Massachusetts it may be found at *Massachusetts General Laws, Chapter 71, Section 55A.* This law applies to public and collaborative school teachers, nurses, principals, and other public or collaborative school employees, and protects them from liability when they provide emergency first aid to a student experiencing a critical medical situation. It also states that the person administering emergency treatment can not be charged monetary expenses if their actions, despite their best efforts, cause the student to be hospitalized, nor can the school employee be the subject of any disciplinary action for responding to the health needs of a student. Good Samaritan laws should help to alleviate the fears of school employees who find themselves in a position where they need to respond to a medical emergency. To find out if your state has a Good Samaritan law, and to determine exactly what it covers, contact a legal professional who can advise you on this.

STATE LAWS WHICH REQUIRE FOOD ALLERGY MANAGEMENT AT SCHOOL

Over the past ten years it has become increasingly clear that food allergies are affecting more and more school-aged children. It has also become clear that accommodations for food-allergic students are very often required in order for them to attend school safely and take full advantage of educational opportunities. Time and experience have demonstrated that school districts benefit when they standardize their approach to food allergy management. In general, having policies that address this issue tends to create less confusion among school staff responsible for implementing procedures meant to minimize a student's risk of experiencing an allergic reaction (see Chapter 4 on District Policy). Recognizing the benefits of food allergy management policy, many states have developed state laws which provide directives to their schools, thus increasing consistency in procedures. Following are examples of four State Departments of Education that have successfully undertaken this task. The information provided summarizes important features of each state law.

The Rhode Island Food Allergy Law (RI 2008 Public Law 08-086)

This law, which was amended in June, 2008, now requires at all school levels, including high school, that:

- for all schools that have an identified student with a peanut and/or tree nut allergy, a notice is posted at all points of entry to the school building, including in the cafeteria, in a conspicuous place.

- each student at risk for anaphylaxis is allowed to carry an epinephrine auto-injector, at all times, when appropriate.

- a medically identified student may self-administer epinephrine auto-injector, if appropriate

This law requires that at the elementary, middle school and junior high school levels:

- policies must be developed which create safe school environments for students with peanut/tree nut allergies.

- Individual Health Care Plans (IHCP) and Emergency Health Care Plans (EHCP) must be developed for each student who has a peanut/tree nut allergy. Accommodations within a peanut/tree nut allergic student's IHCP should include both preventative and emergency measures, and may include, but are not limited to, protocols that:

  ▶ prohibit the sale of particular food items in school

  ▶ prohibit particular foods from certain classrooms or the cafeteria

  ▶ completely prohibit particular food items from the school or school grounds

▶ designate special table(s) in the cafeteria

▶ implement surface and hand washing practices

▶ educate school personnel, students and families about food allergies

- protocols consistent with each student's health plans are implemented while the student is at school and is participating in school-sponsored events.

- all school staff, including substitute teachers, are informed of and understand the Individualized Healthcare Plan and Emergency Health Care Plan of each of their students.

- the use of food allergens in the allergic student's meals, arts and craft projects, educational tools and for incentives, is eliminated.

Although the legal requirements of this law pertain only to peanut and tree nut allergies, and apply predominantly to the elementary, middle school and junior high school levels, the law makes recommendations that school policies be extended to include high schools and that policies include all other potentially serious food allergies, such as dairy, soy, eggs, wheat, fish and shellfish.

New Jersey (P.L. 2007, c.57)

On March 16, 2007, Governor of New Jersey, Jon Corzine, signed into effect a new law addressing food allergy management in public and nonpublic schools. This law mandates that the Department of Education, in conjunction with other medical and professional organizations, establish guidelines for the development of school policies on food allergy management at school. In addition, it requires that guidelines must be implemented which outline training standards for the administration of epinephrine by auto-injector. In response to this, the New Jersey Department of Education, in cooperation with the New Jersey Department of Health and Senior Services, produced a fourteen page document entitled, "Training Protocols for the Emergency Administration of Epinephrine". Of particular significance is the requirement that epinephrine be kept in a secure but unlocked location which is easily accessible to the nurse or anyone designated to administer epinephrine by auto-injector at school or a school-sponsored activity. The law makes clear that this includes school-sponsored events that occur during school and before/after school hours.

There is one unique feature of this law which is worth highlighting. The language of the document requires schools to *recruit* and train school employees as volunteers who will serve as delegates to the nurse in the emergency administration of epinephrine by auto-injector, when the nurse is not available. Although many state regulations require training of delegates for this purpose, it is unusual to find the requirement that they be recruited. We applaud the State of New Jersey for recognizing the importance of actively seeking individuals who will volunteer to serve as a designee to the nurse to administer life-saving medicine in the event that they are needed.

Connecticut (Public Act 05-104)

This law, titled, *An Act concerning food allergies and the prevention of life-threatening incidents in schools*, was approved on June 7, 2005. Similarities and differences exist within its content as compared with the New Jersey and Rhode Island laws previously discussed. Four important requirements have impacted food allergy management in Connecticut schools as a result.

- Similar to New Jersey law, the Connecticut law required the State Department of Education, in conjunction with the State Department of Public Health, to develop guidelines for the management of life-threatening food allergies, with a deadline imposed of January 1, 2006. Connecticut responded to this mandate and produced "Guidelines for Managing

Life-Threatening Food Allergies in Connecticut Schools". In addition, each board of education was required to implement a plan based on the guidelines by July 1, 2006.

- The requirements outlined in the Connecticut law, in general, must be applied to students at the elementary, middle and high school levels.

- Protocols must be implemented in Connecticut schools to avoid exposure to "food allergens", and not just peanuts and tree nuts, which is all that is legally required by the Rhode Island law discussed above.

- Under Connecticut law, schools must have a process to develop individualized health care plans and emergency treatment plans (referred to as "food allergy action plans") for *all* students identified as having life-threatening food allergies, and does not exclude these students who are at the high school level.

New York (Allergy and Anaphylaxis Act of 2007)

Effective January 3, 2007, *The Allergy and Anaphylaxis Management Act of 2007* amended New York *Public Law 2500-H* by adding a new section titled, "Anaphylactic Policy for School Districts". Now referred to as *Public Health Law 2500-H*2*, this new section requires the Commissioner of Health and the Commissioner of Education to establish an anaphylaxis policy for school districts. It mandates that guidelines and procedures be developed for school districts to follow for the prevention and treatment of anaphylaxis. Specifically, the policy is required to establish:

- responsibilities for school nurses and other school personnel as they relate to anaphylaxis management,

- training for the prevention and treatment of anaphylaxis,

- guidelines for the development of emergency tr which are individualized for each student,

- a plan for the communication of related sc and,

- strategies to reduce the risk of exposure to allergens that may cause anaphylaxis.

The Commissioner of Health and the Commissioner of Education were instructed to complete this anaphylaxis policy by June 30, 2008, and forward it to all local school boards of education, charter schools and boards of cooperative educational services. Each entity that receives this policy must review its contents and implement procedures based on its recommendations.

NEW FEDERAL LAW FOR
SCHOOL FOOD ALLERGY MANAGEMENT

S.510 FDA FOOD SAFETY MODERNIZATION ACT
Section 112 Food Allergy and Anaphylaxis Management

A huge step forward has been made toward standardizing school food allergy management with the passage of S.510: FDA Food Safety Modernization Act. This bill was passed by the 111th Congress in the second session and was signed into law by President Obama on January 4, 2011. The Food Allergy and Anaphylaxis Management Act (FAAMA), which was first proposed in 2005, is included in the Food Safety Bill as Section 112. FAAMA directs the US Secretary of Health and Human Services, Kathleen Sebelius, in consultation with the US Secretary of Education, Arne Duncan, to develop and make available national guidelines for the management of food allergy and anaphylaxis at school. Once developed, these guidelines may be adopted on a voluntary basis by public schools. In addition, schools that choose to implement the recommended procedures will be eligible for food allergy management grants. Eligibility to receive grant money will require the school to complete and submit an application to the US Secretary of Health and Human Services. The duration of a grant awarded to a school will be no longer than two years, and a grant awarded under this subsection may not be made in an amount that is more than $50,000.00 annually.

Areas to be addressed in the federal guidelines will include:

1. The parent's obligation in the management of their child's food allergy while at school,

2. "The creation and maintenance of an individual plan for management of the student's food allergy(s), in consultation with the parent, tailored to the needs of each child with a documented risk for anaphylaxis . . .",

3. Communication strategies between the school and providers of emergency medical services,

4. Strategies to reduce the risk of exposure to the student's allergens in the classroom and in common areas of the school, such as the cafeteria,

5. General education about food allergies provided for school staff, parents and students,

6. Training and education on food allergy management provided to school personnel who have regular contact with students who have life threatening allergies,

7. Training and authorization of school personnel to administer epinephrine by auto-injector when the school nurse is not readily available,

8. Timely access to epinephrine by auto-injector by school personnel when the school nurse is not immediately available,

9. Development of an individual plan to treat an incident of anaphylaxis should it occur during school-sponsored extra-curricular or before and after school activities, or field trips,

10. Information and record-keeping for each administration of epinephrine to a student who has experienced anaphylaxis, including timely notification to the child's parents.

The US Secretary of Health and Human Services has one year from the date of the bill's signing to develop these national guidelines. Recommendations included in these national guidelines will not be intended to supersede state laws. It should be noted that the Food Allergy and Anaphylaxis Network was instrumental in championing efforts to get this legislation passed.

PENDING FEDERAL LEGISLATION: "SCHOOL ACCESS EMERGENCY EPINEPHRINE ACT"

A national initiative is underway to pass legislation which would provide an incentive for states to adopt laws that would allow schools to have a "stock" supply of epinephrine auto-injectors readily available. These epinephrine auto-injectors, such as the EpiPen®, could be used on any student or staff who experiences anaphylaxis in the school setting. This bill was introduced to the U.S. Senate (S.1884) on November 12, 2011, by Senators Dick Durbin (D-IL) and Mark Kirk (R-IL). It was then introduced to the House a month later on December 8, 2011, (H.R. 3627), by Representative Phil Roe (R-TN) and Democratic Whip Steny Hoyer (D-MD).

The bill references pertinent information reported by The National Institute of Allergy and Infectious Diseases (NIAID) which states that prompt administration of epinephrine to treat anaphylaxis is critical to a positive outcome, and that a delay in receiving epinephrine can result in death. Study results indicate that 25% of incidents of anaphylaxis at school involve individuals with no previous history of severe allergy. A school physician can provide what are called "standing orders" for epinephrine auto-injectors to be on hand at school, so that any student or staff member, including those who do not have their own physician-prescribed epinephrine, may be treated with this life-saving medicine should they experience an anaphylactic event. Passage of this legislation would be a significant step forward in helping to prevent allergy-related deaths.

This legislation has been brought to the forefront by the Food Allergy and Anaphylaxis Network, and is supported and endorsed by the American Academy of Allergy, Asthma and Immunology (AAAAI), the American College of Allergy, Asthma and Immunology (ACAAI), the American Academy of Pediatrics (AAP), the National Association of Elementary School Principals (NAESP), the National Association of School Nurses (NASN) and the American Academy of Emergency Medicine (AAEM).

Conclusion

In summary, the best approach to address the needs of a food-allergic student, and also be in compliance with relevant laws, would be to:

- Have a general understanding of the civil rights and special education laws discussed in this chapter,

- Ensure that the student with a food allergy has a healthcare plan that adequately meets the requirements stated in these federal and state laws and also meets the student's special health needs,

- Educate and train school staff to understand the nature of food allergies, how to prevent allergic reactions from happening, and how to treat a reaction should one occur.

Knowledge, care, and planning will greatly contribute to the goal of keeping students with food allergies safe while at school. The Massachusetts Department of Public Health, in the publication, **The Comprehensive School Health Manual**, sums up the many benefits of such an approach by saying, "Thoughtful planning for students with special health care needs promotes quality school-based care, helps to insure that these students are able to participate to the fullest possible extent in educational and social opportunities, and minimizes the potential for liability, which may be a concern of many school personnel". I couldn't agree more!

Important Points to Remember

▶ A life-threatening food allergy meets the definition of a disability as determined by the United States Department of Education's Office for Civil Rights. Therefore, a student with a physician-documented life-threatening food allergy is entitled to protection under federal law, such as Section 504 of the Rehabilitation Act of 1973.

▶ No child may be refused admittance to a school or program based on a disability. Period. This is in violation of civil rights laws.

▶ Students may not be excluded or segregated from the classroom curriculum, including extra-curricular activities, and before or after school activities based on their disability. This includes the cafeteria, field trips, and school-sponsored sports and recreational events.

▶ Students with food allergies may not be excluded from the public school lunch program if they choose to buy lunch. Accommodations must be made to insure safe and equal participation in the school lunch program, at no extra cost to the family.

▶ Schools have a duty to care for all their students. Therefore, liability waivers that ignore this requirement should not be requested of parents (and if requested, should not be signed by parents).

▶ Federal laws take precedence over conflicting state and local laws.

▶ Even if there is not a full-time nurse at your child's school, your child is entitled to reliable administration of physician-ordered medicine. Parents may not be required to administer medication to their child at school.

Information included in this chapter should not be considered legal advice for any specific situation. Any questions should be directed to a competent legal professional for counsel and advice.

SUPPLEMENTAL MATERIALS

SCHOOLS, FOOD ALLERGIES AND THE LAWS

Schools have a responsibility to provide a safe environment for all children while providing the resources and opportunities necessary for them to thrive educationally. It is critical that school staff understand the federal and state laws which protect students who have life-threatening food allergies as they strive to meet these goals. Special attention should be paid to the following three federal laws: the Rehabilitation Act of 1973, Section 504, the Americans with Disabilities Act of 1990 (ADA), and the Individuals with Disabilities Education Act (IDEA).

The Rehabilitation Act of 1973, Section 504 is enforced by the U.S. Department of Education, Office for Civil Rights (OCR), and was constructed to "prohibit discrimination on the basis of disability in education . . . in any program or institution receiving federal funds . . ." Under Section 504, a person is defined as having a disability if one or more life activities are substantially limited. The OCR formally defines life-threatening food allergies as a disability. Section 504 does not have federal or state funding to assist districts to meet obligations in complying with implementation of its accommodations. *Children with physician—documented, life-threatening food allergies are eligible to receive accommodations under a "504 Plan" which defines procedures to keep the student safe while at school. What this means to educators is that modifications may need to be made to classroom programs and materials in order to meet the special needs of these students.*

The Americans With Disabilities Act of 1990 (ADA), enforced by the U.S. Department of Justice, states that " . . . no individual shall be discriminated against on the basis of disability in the full and equal enjoyment of the goods (and) services . . . of any . . . public accommodation . . ." Public accommodation means that schools must make sure "that no individual with a disability is excluded, denied services, segregated, or otherwise treated differently than other individuals because of the absence of auxiliary aids and services." Title II of the ADA addresses individuals with disabilities in state and local government agencies and programs, such as public schools. Title III addresses places of public accommodation whether or not they receive federal funds. Private schools and preschools would fall under this category. *School staff must provide educational activities which allow disabled students to participate in programs offered safely and without segregation.*

The Individuals with Disabilities Education Act (IDEA), enforced by the U.S. Department of Education, Office of Special Education & Rehabilitative Services, was written to ensure that children with disabilities receive the services necessary " . . . to allow them to benefit from their educational program." This statute has thirteen designations for disabilities and allows for financial assistance to states for services for students with these disabilities. *Under IDEA, the concept of a school's "duty to care" for all students, includes written plans and strategies intended to enable the child to meet their educational goals. This often takes the form of an Individualized Educational Program, or IEP, if special education teacher instruction services are needed.*

For more specific information regarding the laws and regulations which protect the rights of children with food allergies, contact an attorney and/or a competent food allergy consultant. The U.S. Departments of Justice and Education may be contacted, as well as individual State and local Departments of Education and Public Health.

LIFE-THREATENING FOOD ALLERGIES
AND
SECTION 504 PLAN ELIGIBILITY

The U.S. Office for Civil Rights (OCR), U.S. Department of Education, formally recognizes *allergy* as a "hidden disability". The OCR defines hidden disabilities as "physical or mental impairments that are not readily apparent to others." The physical or mental impairment must substantially limit one or more major life activities. The physiological condition of food allergy may affect the respiratory, digestive, cardiovascular and skin body systems. An individual with a life-threatening food allergy could experience difficulty breathing and a severe drop in blood pressure during an anaphylactic reaction. Therefore, life-threatening food allergies meet the definition of qualifying impairments under Section 504 of the Rehabilitation Act of 1973.

Once a school (which is a recipient of federal funds from the U.S. Department of Education) receives a request for a student to have protection under Section 504, a meeting should be scheduled to determine the student's eligibility for this protection. Documentation from the child's physician which verifies the diagnosis of the student's life-threatening food allergy should be presented. If the student's health meets the qualifications for protection under Section 504, the school has a legal obligation to provide the appropriate services to meet the special needs of that student.

Source: Pamphlet: *"The Civil Rights of Students with Hidden Disabilities Under Section 504 of the Rehabilitation Act of 1973"*

U.S. Department of Education, Office for Civil Rights

www2.ed.gov/about/offices/list/OCR/docs/hq5269.html

SECTION 504 vs. IDEA

Section 504	**IDEA**
Section 504 of the Rehabilitation Act of 1973	Individuals with Disabilities Education Act
Civil Rights Law—protects rights of disabled individuals	Federal statute to provide aid to states for students with disabilities
Enforced by: US Dept. of Ed., Office for Civil Rights (OCR)	Enforced by: US Dept. of Ed., Special Ed. & Rehabilitative Services
Eligibility: physical or mental impairment resulting in substantial limitation of 1 or more life activities (example: breathing)	Eligibility: 13 formal disability designations—autism, deaf-blindness, emotional disturbance, hearing impairment, mental retardation, multiple disabilities, orthopedic impairment, other health impairment, specific learning disability, speech or language impairment, traumatic brain injury, visual impairment, including blindness
Disability falls under Section 504 if it does not require special education teacher instructional services	**Disability falls under IDEA if it does require special education teacher instructional services**

Section 504	**IDEA**
Example: food allergies, asthma that does not affect learning	Example: acute asthma that affects learning (under "other health impairment")
Managed by: Sec. 504 Coordinator, Nurse	Managed by: Special Ed. Department
Accommodation: "504 Plan"	Accommodation: "IEP"
Students entitled to a "Free Appropriate Education" (FAPE)	Students entitled to a "Free Appropriate Education" (FAPE)
Evaluation: requires parental notice and periodic re-evaluation	Evaluation: requires consent for initial evaluation at a minimum, once every three years
Parent Notification: notice regarding identification, evaluation or placement	Parent Notification: written notice re. identification, evaluation or placement
Planning: parents are not required to be part of the planning team, and their signature on the "504 Plan" is NOT required	Planning: parents are required to be part of the planning team and their signature IS required on the "IEP"
Due Process Rights: requires impartial hearing	Due Process Rights: requires impartial hearing
Grievance: requires designation by district compliance officer and formal procedure	Grievance: NO required grievance procedure or Compliance officer

Section 504	**IDEA**
Funding: NO federal funds	Funding: Receives federal funds called "Federal Financial Assistance" or "FFA's"; for a school to be eligible to receive FFA's, they must comply with Section 504 regulations and requirements.

Note: Schools determine whether a disability falls under Section 504 or IDEA by looking at the acuteness of the disability (the definition of "disability" is broader under Section 504 than that found in the IDEA), and is fact-specific. Whenever there is a question, contact a legal consultant knowledgeable in this area.

ACCOMMODATIONS FOR STUDENTS WITH SPECIAL DIETARY NEEDS

Here is important information all school personnel and parents of children with life-threatening food allergies should know when the decision is made to have a food-allergic student buy lunch in the school cafeteria:

The U.S. Department of Agriculture, Food and Nutrition Service, offers guidance to schools and specifically school food service staff, to meet the requirements of children with special dietary needs, in accordance with federal regulation 7 CFR 15b (USDA). The publication is entitled:

"ACCOMMODATING CHILDREN WITH SPECIAL DIETARY NEEDS IN THE SCHOOL NUTRITION PROGRAMS"

RESPONSIBILITY OF THE FAMILY

If a family has a child with life-threatening food allergies, and chooses to have the child buy lunch, the parents must submit documentation to the school, signed by their physician, which explains:

1. The disability and why it restricts their diet,

2. The major life activity affected (i.e., eating), and

3. The food or foods to be omitted and the foods to be used as substitutions.

RESPONSIBILITY OF THE SCHOOL

1. Staff is required to prepare safe meals of equivalent nutritional value if requested by the family of the student with life-threatening food allergies, and

2. This special meal must be provided at no extra cost to the family.

Families should meet with school food service staff well in advance, in order that the school may have sufficient time to adequately meet the special needs of the child with food allergies.

FOR MORE SPECIFIC INFORMATION, REFER TO:

USDA, FOOD AND NUTRITION SERVICES

FNS INSTRUCTION 783-2, REVISION 2

"MEAL SUBSTITUTIONS FOR MEDICAL OR OTHER SPECIAL DIETARY REASONS"

OR: Contact the Child and Nutrition Program located in your State Department of Education

"Optimism is the faith that leads to achievement
be done without hope and confidenc

Helen Keller

CHAPTER FIVE

THE IMPACT OF FOOD ALLERGIES: WORKING THROUGH THE EMOTIONS

When working with children who have food allergies, the focus is most often on efforts and strategies which address keeping these children safe from physical harm. This is obviously appropriate. However, an area which is often overlooked is the impact living with food allergies has on the child. For students, school policies must be in place that address the student's physical *and* emotional health. This chronic health condition must be safely navigated by the student on a daily basis, and that can at times, take its toll. It should be no surprise that the lives of other members of the food-allergic child's family will also be affected. A 2004 study which looked specifically at the quality of life experienced by families of children with food allergies found that all members of these families undergo a plethora of emotions.

How the *child* with food allergies might be affected.

Children with food allergies certainly need to deal with the challenges presented to them as a result of having a food allergy. Many of these youngsters seem able to understand how serious it is to have a food allergy at a very young age. Lisa Cipriano Collins, who wrote, _Caring for Your Child with Severe Food Allergies,_ says that a child with food allergies " . . . is robbed of a carefree childhood and instead must be careful and responsible before his/her time." That is not to say that children with food allergies will not encounter fun and enjoyable experiences in their lives. What it does mean, however, is that a child with a food allergy will need to approach many situations differently than most of his/her peers. The process to allow for fun is more involved and detail-oriented. Each activity must be assessed from the standpoint of "Will this be safe for me?" Children may respond to the feelings this provokes in many different ways.

Some children with food allergies may react with feelings of anger and frustration and believe that having a food allergy is "unfair". It is not easy to accept the fact that certain foods that look interesting and appealing may not be eaten. It is also difficult to accept that many activities may not be attended with the same carefree-abandon as by children without food allergies. Fun activities that are hallmarks of youth, such as birthday parties, holiday celebrations, play dates and outings to the park or playground must be researched by the parents and approached only after safety precautions have been put into place. Although the young child with a food allergy does not personally do this advance planning, he or she may sense the tension, and at times the fatigue, that this endeavor may provoke in the parent who is doing the planning. Furthermore, these children are often given specific instructions before attending the "fun" activity, such as reminders to wash their hands, check with an adult before eating any treats, and know where their EpiPen® will be kept. These instructions, though necessary, may instill a sense of uneasiness in the child, which in turn, may also deflate some of the joy and excitement. There are other social situations in which children with food allergies are completely left out because they may not be able to participate safely at all. Going to the ice cream or pizza parlor may not be an option for the child with a dairy allergy, and an outing to the baseball park may never be a reality for children with peanut allergies. It is easy to understand that this may, at times, make the child with food allergies feel angry, frustrated, resentful and sad.

Another scenario which provokes similar feelings is when the child with a food allergy becomes the victim of hurtful remarks made by a peer or classmate who chooses to reference their food allergy in negative and demeaning terms. Teasing and taunting a child with comments such as, "Too bad you can't eat this peanut butter and jelly sandwich—it's so good!" are difficult to hear. The emotional pain felt by children who have been subjected to physical threats to their safety, is surely profound. In addition to feeling angry, frustrated and sad, the child on the receiving end of these bullying words or actions is also left to feel embarrassed and perhaps ashamed that they are somehow "different" than "normal" kids. No one wants to be singled out in this way, and to say that these experiences cause pain and suffering would be an understatement. School personnel must take threats of harassment seriously and put an end to them immediately before they escalate into situations of real physical harm to the student. A school nurse or principal can greatly reduce these negative behaviors by providing peer and parent education on food allergies to the school community. Most people, both young and old, will be more willing to help protect a child with food allergies when they have a better understanding of the life-threatening nature of this health condition and the far reaching ways in which it impacts the child's everyday life.

How children respond to difficult frustrations related to their food allergies will depend on many factors such as their age, temperament, maturity, etc. The ways in which family members handle troublesome situations may also influence their response and attitude. Some children by nature are not easily shaken and are able to take things in relative stride. Some children may be outwardly demonstrative and deal with feelings of anger by exhibiting aggressive behaviors, such as shouting or acting out towards their siblings, peers, or parents. Others may be more passive and reticent in their approach, while others may quietly cry tears of frustration.

Children with food allergies may also become anxious and fearful over the possibility of having a reaction, especially if they have had one that they are old enough to remember. They may worry and seem nervous at the prospect of what they view as an unsafe situation or activity. They may be hesitant about things that, at first glance, seem unrelated to their food allergy. For example, some children with food allergies who are particularly anxious may demonstrate a reluctance to go to a friend's house, particularly if it is for the first time, or to ride the school bus or to take part in any new experience, for that matter. They may not be able to express verbally that their reticence is most likely due to a fear of the unknown. Their home is a safe and controlled environment, while the outside world does not offer this same level of confidence. Without this sense of familiarity and resulting comfort, life may seem open to too many risks with potentially harmful consequences. As a result, it is not uncommon for children with food allergies to prefer keeping as many routines as a part of their daily life as possible. They may have difficulty accepting any change to their routine because this makes them feel susceptible to risks. An unexpected adjustment to a schedule, such as having art class on a school day which doesn't ordinarily have art, may cause feelings of uneasiness and stress.

In addition to a having a propensity for routines, children with food allergies may develop control issues over food. Food, by necessity, must be approached with caution. Therefore, some children may prefer to eat the same foods over, and over, and over again, because their history with these foods has demonstrated that they are safe. For example, it may be important for a child with food allergies that his/her lunch is made of the exact same items every day for long periods of time. Any change to the "status quo" may result in an emotional protest. What is important is that the assortment of foods the child chooses to eat will allow for a balanced diet which meets all nutritional needs.

According to allergist Scott Sicherer, MD, some children with severe food allergies may develop psychosomatic reactions as a result of their worry and anxiety. It is important to understand that fear and anxiety can cause real physical symptoms. For example, even if no allergen has been ingested, the overwhelming fear of having eaten something to which a child is allergic may trigger a panic attack in that child. He or she may experience such things as an itchy throat, difficulty breathing, light headedness, etc. A panic attack may produce symptoms that closely mimic the symptoms of an allergic reaction. Another example of a psychosomatic reaction would be when a child believes symptoms of an allergic reaction are being experienced after having eaten a food previously tolerated. Dr. Sicherer defines this as a "generalization of reactions" when these reported symptoms can not be attributed to the development of a new allergy. In extreme cases, phobias related to food and eating have contributed to eating disorders in some children with food allergies. If you suspect that a child is experiencing psychosomatic symptoms and/or phobias regarding his/her food allergy, it would be important to seek the help and advice of a physician or psychologist as soon as possible.

Similarly to other children with chronic health conditions, children with food allergies may develop feelings of sadness. This response is usually short-lived, however if a child remains sad for an extended period of time, it may signal clinical depression. Symptoms of depression may be seen as a prolonged and unexplained fatigue, a lack of interest or a significant decrease in doing activities which were previously enjoyed and valued, a change in sleeping patterns, such as either needing too much sleep or not being able to sleep easily, or feelings of worthlessness. If these symptoms become noticeable and persist and cause concern, then it would be advisable to seek professional help. A pediatrician or perhaps the school psychologist would be good resources in this type of situation. Other parents of children with food allergies can also be a source of support and information.

It is generally recognized that food allergy may negatively impact quality of life. This may be particularly true for teenagers with a diagnosis of food allergy. In a study reported in November, 2010, researchers developed a validated quality of life questionnaire designed specifically to address this issue for food-allergic teenagers in the United States. Not surprisingly, analysis of the answers given by 203 participants aged 13-19 years demonstrates that these young people experience notable difficulties with social and emotional issues. Areas cited as causing most concern for these adolescents were limitations on social activities and choice of restaurants, as well as an inability to eat the same foods as others. Participants in the study also expressed concern over the belief that their schools do not provide sufficient education about food allergies to members of their school community. Lower quality of life scores were found in adolescents with a history of anaphylaxis, as compared with those who did not have a history of anaphylaxis.

It is safe to say that the teenage years present a particularly complicated time for the child with food allergies. In general, when students enter high school, they are entering a time in their lives where they need and very often crave more independence. Most children at this age desire more control over their lives and have a marked decrease in their desire for parental input and involvement. It is safe to say that starting now, friendships rule and parents/adults drool! This is a time when children are more likely to partake in risk taking behaviors. Practical reasoning takes a backseat, and life is approached with emotion as the driving force. The need to fit in and not be "different" intensifies. Teenagers also tend to feel and react to things on a grandiose scale, and often have extreme responses to their world. When their world includes having a food allergy, another layer is added to the already difficult social arena that they are experiencing developmentally at this time. This can cause unique complications for the teen with a food allergy. Coupled with a sense of being "invincible" at this time, a youngster who has not had an allergic reaction over a considerable period of time, may convince him or herself that the food allergy has been outgrown. Serious ramifications may result if this denial leads to such risk taking behaviors as eating foods without checking for safe ingredients, and participating in social activities without having potentially life-saving medicines on hand, such as the EpiPen®.

A discussion describing how a child might be affected by food allergy would not be complete without including the fact that positive responses are also very possible. These youngsters often take on responsibilities typical of an older child due to the necessity of keeping themselves safe. As a result, it is not unusual for young children with a food allergy to behave with impressive maturity. A child with food allergies may also have a tendency to be introspective and contemplative in his/her approach to life. Many children with food allergies also seem to have a sense of empathy regarding the differences in all of us and easily demonstrate caring and kindness towards others. These are certainly desirable traits, and this positive response to learning to live with a food allergy is one which we need to recognize and appreciate.

How *brothers and sisters* of the child with food allergies might be affected.

Siblings of a child with food allergies may also experience a sense of fear, although in this case, the fear is born out of concern for the health and safety of their brother or sister. They are not immune to worrying about the wellbeing of their food-allergic sibling and very often may find themselves in this state of mind. Guilt is another emotion that may be felt by a sibling of a child with food allergies. These children may find themselves feeling guilty that they don't have a food allergy, out of a sense of empathy for their sibling. Conversely, they may also feel guilty because they are, in fact, glad that they don't have a food allergy. This can be a difficult mix of emotions to understand and reconcile. Siblings might be envious of the "special" attention received by their brother or sister who has food allergies. It is easy to feel left out and perhaps even unimportant when their mom or dad is spending so much time with their sibling with food allergies. They also may be resentful that certain foods aren't allowed in the house, especially if the banished foods are ones which they enjoy. Difficulties can arise when these feelings and emotions are not addressed.

How the *parents* might be affected.

Most parents feel a sense of shock when they hear the diagnosis of a "life-threatening food allergy" given to their loved one. These words tend to send minds whirling and hearts pounding. An immediate response might be to believe that this simply can not be true. To say that it is difficult to grasp and fully understand the full meaning of this diagnosis when it is first given is an understatement.

Lisa Cipriano Collins believes that the foremost emotion experienced by parents of children with food allergies is **STRESS**. Stress is capable of causing physical, mental or emotional pain. Most parents of children with food allergies would agree that it is not an easy endeavor when caring for a child who may suffer life-threatening consequences from eating an infinitesimal amount of food. The challenges are many and parents find themselves exerting constant care and attention to every detail in order to keep their child out of harm's way. These parents must *always* plan ahead, and contemplate all imaginable variables required to ensure a safe outing. Ingredients of foods to be eaten by their child need to be checked in advance, the EpiPen® and any other related medicines must be remembered whenever leaving the house, arrangements for "safe" foods are made when necessary, vital and possibly life-saving information must be explained to caregivers, and the list goes on. This constant attention to minute but critically important details can be draining both physically and emotionally. Parents describe feeling "on edge", "on alert", "on guard", etc., a great deal of the time, especially when leaving the house. No stone is left unturned, at least not knowingly, and the pressures of this responsibility are enormous. The result can be an overwhelming and persistent sense of fatigue.

The emotions parents feel as a result of this stress may be manifested in a variety of ways: *Fear, Anxiety, Guilt, Anger, Frustration, Confusion, and Sadness,* for example.

Parents may experience the unsettling pangs of anxiety and fear that their child may have an allergic reaction, despite their best efforts, on a regular basis. These are feelings which tend to persist throughout each day, every day. Parents can be consumed by this constant worry, which may give them little time and energy to devote to other concerns, interests or the needs of other family members or themselves. The realization that other areas of their life are being under-addressed can be a catalyst for feelings of guilt. Some parents have also expressed feelings of guilt for a totally different reason. They believe that they may be responsible for their child's food allergy based on some previous activity, such as eating peanut butter during pregnancy or during the period of time that their child was breastfed. It is important to understand that no studies to date offer clear evidence to support this belief. These feelings, however, are based deeply in emotion, and they may result in a heavy sense of often unspoken guilt.

Parents may feel angry that their child has a food allergy. The realization that a loved one will go through life facing the frightening prospect of experiencing a severe allergic reaction can be difficult to bear. Parents may feel frustrated that they can't change this diagnosis for their child. Parents may also experience confusion as to how they might best manage their child's food allergy, for the sake of their child and their family. This type of confusion can also lead to feelings of frustration. Parents may feel sadness that their child may not have the same childhood experiences that are traditionally enjoyed by other children (pizza parties, ball games, ice cream parlors, for example), and sadness once it is understood that this diagnosis will now change the ways in which all involved will conduct their lives.

Parents experience these myriad emotions with repetitive fluidity. In other words, there may be much movement in emotions over the course of one day, and from day to day, depending on encounters and experiences. One moment a parent may be happy about how a situation was handled, and the next day, after a close encounter with an offending allergen, or an unkind remark, feelings of fear, anger, worry and sadness may be brought to the forefront. Everyone brings different personalities to the table, and this too, will affect the ways in which a person reacts to each situation with which he or she is faced.

Can having a child with food allergies cause *conflict between the parents*?

Simply put, yes, it may. I have worked with families where the parents were not in agreement as to how their child's food allergies should be managed, and this conflict caused many stressful feelings for each of the parents. It is possible for one parent to be more casual, maybe even a little laidback, in his/her approach to managing their child's food allergy. This style may be uncomfortable for the other parent, who may be fastidious and methodical in handling their child's food allergy. Heated discussions may ensue over whether or not it is necessary, for example, to bring the EpiPen® wherever their child will travel, regardless of whether food will be eaten. The statement, *"But he's not going to be eating anything!"* may be a regular source of conflict. How can two individuals react to the same situation in two totally different ways? The answer is partly found in the definition of the word, "individual". As human beings, we are each distinct entities, complete with our own particular attributes and identifying traits. We each bring to the table our own individual personalities, backgrounds and experiences. Given this dynamic, it becomes possible to understand how each parent may perceive their child's food allergy, and how it should be managed, in different ways.

These differing perspectives, perceptions and approaches can, over time, cause resentment, frustration, and difficulties. Clear, calm communication between the parents would be a good way to keep these types of conflicts to a minimum. Each parent should have the opportunity to explain their point of view, and expect to be heard with as much of an open mind as is humanly possible. The most productive discussions are usually those which are kept relatively unemotional, although this may be admittedly, difficult to do. Written information which helps to support a particular opinion could be shared during this time. The bottom line is that ultimately, both parents need to understand that their *child's safety needs to be the foremost concern,* and that taking any chances where this is concerned would not make good sense. Working differences out privately and with the goal of reaching a shared approach which doesn't risk giving mixed messages is important. Contributing to your child's confusion as to how his/her food allergy should be managed is definitely not a desirable outcome. Counseling is always an option if, despite best efforts, a reasonable sense of "being on the same page" cannot be reached.

COPING STRATEGIES

To Keep You Moving Forward

For the Parents

Some parents are able to successfully manage the stress they feel in order to meet these daily challenges. They are adept in not letting their feelings negatively affect their behavior and health, or that of their family's, including their food-allergic child. Many parents, however, find they have some level of difficulty managing these rather complicated emotions on a regular basis. It is important for parents to develop a sense of acceptance and develop a healthy approach to managing their child's food allergy in a manner which works for themselves, their child, and for the rest of their family. In order to move forward in a positive and productive manner, the following are some strategies and practical suggestions meant to assist parents in dealing effectively with the myriad emotions that life with a food allergy will likely provoke. The overall goal in managing a child's food allergy is to find ways to keep the child safe while also trying to keep all lives involved as normal and relaxed (the antonym to "stress"!) as possible.

First: Understand that if you have experienced any or all of the emotions discussed earlier, anxiety, fear, guilt, sadness, etc., that you are not alone! It is o.k. to feel these emotions and most parents of children with food allergies certainly have. You may need to allow yourself to experience these feelings in order to ***move forward***. Fear, when kept in check, can actually help you make good decisions by allowing you to proceed with caution and forethought. Parents of children with food allergies *must* proceed with extreme care as they attempt to avoid allergens and allergic reactions. When does fear advance to a place where it is no longer productive? Fear becomes unreasonable when it is so extensive that it makes you feel paralyzed, you are not able to make a decision, and you find yourself saying "No" to everything.

Second: Try and understand that while you might have numerous and varied emotions, what is *important is how you manage these feelings*. It is important to work with your emotions constructively. Guilt is a particularly non-productive emotion: *it does no one any good*. It is important to push it aside so that you may ***move forward***. Feelings of fear and despair can sometimes be managed by approaching them from a perspective of logical thinking, rather than emotion. If you are anxious about the safety of a social event, take a step back, assess the situation and approach it from a practical standpoint: What are the risks? What are the benefits? Are there steps you can take to make the situation reasonably safe for your child? How important is the event to your child? Based on your analysis, some events will be attended, and some events will be missed. This is o.k. This is life. Make a decision based on your evaluation of the facts, and ***move forward.***

If you are feeling angry at the reaction of another person regarding your child's food allergies, for example if a person has been insensitive or rude in a remark, or perhaps has been unwilling to help or cooperate in some way, the best approach is to try to educate this individual in a non-preaching and calm manner. Many people "don't get it" because they really don't understand what true food allergies are all about. It is possible, however, that some "nay sayers" will never get it. Try and accept the fact that some people, despite your best efforts, *will never get it.* Focus on those who understand and are willing to help so that you can ***move forward***.

I believe that an important key in reducing your stress and anxiety is when you are able to identify those situations which provoke high amounts of stress for you. When you are able to recognize and understand the causes of your stress, you may then work to figure out what can be done to reduce your stress. Through both my personal and professional experiences with families, I have found that transitional times tend to be the cause of significant stress for families of children with food allergies. Entering preschool, kindergarten or any new school, such as going from elementary school to middle school, can be quite difficult. Parents often experience a tremendous amount of anxiety over the question of whether their child will be safe in this new environment, and if so, how. This concern is obviously understandable. The best way to handle these feelings and help insure that there will be safe practices in place, would be to do your homework so that you can be prepared.

At school, have an approach that would be considered professional and positive. Samuel Johnson was quoted as saying, "Clear you mind of 'can't'." Adopt this as a motto and remember that this is a process. Each step forward is a success and even a small success is still a success! Help prepare staff by educating them on food allergies and ways to reduce a child's risk of exposure to his/her allergens. Get to know the "players", such as the nurse, principal, teacher, etc. and become familiar with the school environment. Learn about the current procedures being implemented to manage food allergies at the school, such as hand washing practices, whether or not there are sinks in the classrooms, if allergens are allowed in the areas where your child will travel, the location of the EpiPen® and who is trained to administer it, etc. Work with school staff to develop practical avoidance strategies to be written into your child's Individual Healthcare Plan.

Parents who get involved with the Parent-Teacher Organization (PTO) find this to be extremely helpful in their efforts to 1.) become knowledgeable about events being planned for the school community and 2.) develop relationships with other parents and school personnel who have decision-making responsibilities as they pertain to these events. Without a doubt, when you plan ahead, you will be better prepared to advocate for your child's health and safety, and this will add to your feelings of confidence in the likelihood of achieving this desired outcome.

If you find yourself meeting roadblocks, having a bad day, or hitting a rough patch, find out what works best for you to lower and manage your stress. Simple practices that are calming often can be very helpful. Listening to music, taking a hot bath, watching a comedy, going for a walk, taking some quiet time just for you in order to "regroup", might be exactly what is needed. The goal is to work through the emotions, so that you can *move forward.*

Third: Keep yourself educated about food allergies and recommended management strategies. Make sure **you** are fully educated and informed about your child's allergy. You are, after all, your child's best advocate. Ask your doctor to explain food allergies and the ways in which your child may be exposed to the offending allergens. Discuss the proper use and storage of the EpiPen® and the ways which are recommended to treat an allergic reaction for your child. You should also have your allergist help you prepare a written treatment plan intended as your child's "Emergency Treatment Plan" (ETP), which will need to be followed by the school nurse or your child's teachers, should your child experience an allergic reaction while at school.

Find out and become a member of local and national support groups. The Asthma and Allergy Foundation of America and The Food Allergy and Anaphylaxis Network are recommended and can be great sources of important information. Use any materials that are offered from these groups to help increase your arsenal of knowledge. Tal with families of other children with food allergies to share helpful information. Ideas shared in this way can be invaluable and also save you precious time. An added benefit is that talking with other people who truly "get it" gives you the opportunity to vent, helps you to validate your feelings and know that you are not alone, and gives you the information and support that is so important and necessary.

The more informed you are, the easier it is to make better decisions. When you take control of the situation, you also put yourself in a better place to take control of your emotions. Very simply put, let yourself experience your feelings and emotions, but don't let them consume you. Help yourself to work through them by taking a practical approach to managing your child's food allergies. Adopting a process of rational and systematic thought, along with an attitude that you *can* work through this, will help you to keep *moving forward*.

For the Sibling of your Food-Allergic Child

If the scenarios discussed earlier regarding how the sibling of a food-allergic child might feel sound familiar, it would be important to let your child without food allergies know that you understand. It is often very helpful to talk candidly about why things are being done the way they are, so that a better understanding may be reached as to why decisions are being made. Equally important is listening to them so that they may have the opportunity to express their feelings. Communication, understanding and caring can go a long way in ameliorating what can be a difficult and complicated situation. Planning "special" time with these children very often helps them to reaffirm that they are important to you, which, in turn, may result in fewer of these negative feelings from developing. This approach will also aid in fostering their acceptance of circumstances *as they are and need to be*.

l with Food Allergies

goal is to create an environment that is fundamentally
ws for your child to participate, whenever possible, in
normal childhood experiences. As parents, it is our job to help
our children work through the various stages of their development,
whether or not they have a food allergy. Lisa Cipriano Collins points
out that noted psychologist Erik Erikson**, as he wrote in __Childhood
and Society,__** believes that the first stage of development we must
foster in our children is "trust". Therefore, one of the most important
things you can do to help your child cope with having a food allergy
is to work with your child to develop a strong sense of *trust* in his/
her ability to be safe.

When your child is very young, and dependent on you for most
things, it is important for you to help your child develop trust *in
you*. Your toddler, who has not yet acquired the skills of speech, and
who certainly can not read ingredient labels, must rely on you, your
judgment and your efforts to stay safe. Your child needs to trust and
believe in your ability to do this. It is extremely helpful to keep your
communications with your child, as it pertains to his/her food allergy,
in as much of an unemotional and matter-of-fact manner as possible.
If you are feeling extremely nervous, it is important to try and not
communicate this to your child in your words, your mannerisms or
in your facial expressions. Children are perceptive, and they can
often pick up on subtleties of feelings. When you maintain a sense of
outward calm and confidence, even if you are feeling a little shaky
inside, you will help your young child view having a food allergy
from more of a practical standpoint, rather than an emotional one.

As your child gets older, your second focus should be on helping
him or her to feel safe outside of the home. In order to make this
happen, parents need to help their child with food allergies develop
a sense of trust *in other people*, beyond Mom and Dad. This may be
a difficult task if you, as a parent, are having difficulty trusting other
adults to safely care for your child. Once again, a practical approach

is recommended. Work with caregivers in an effort to educate them about how to manage your child's food allergy. Teach them about the procedures necessary to avoid possible allergic reactions and how to treat them should one occur. This will help you to feel more confident about their ability to keep your child safe.

The third focus in this process is for you to help your child believe and trust in *his/her own ability* to keep safe. This is a critical achievement necessary in helping your child to successfully manage his/her allergies and be on the path to becoming a capable, confident and independent person. You need to somehow navigate the fine line between letting your child know how serious having a food allergy is without scaring your child to the point where he or she becomes petrified and is unable to function. Although not an easy task, you want to help your child with food allergies become careful and cautious, not fearful and frantic. Understand that achieving this balance can be difficult. Ways to deal with this challenge may be found in the results of a 2009 study led by Jennifer LeBovidge, Ph.D., of Children's Hospital, Boston, which assessed psychological distress felt by children and teenagers with food allergies. This study found that children's attitudes about their food allergies, such as whether they focus on limitations or differences, or on strengths and coping strategies, were related to emotions such as anxiety or sadness. Parents can ask simple questions aimed at revealing the extent to which they feel different from their peers or limited from participating in activities, to determine whether any issues of concern exist. Children who seem to focus on their limitations and differences may be helped by fostering in them a more positive approach to managing their food allergy. Help them to develop problem-solving skills as they relate to their food allergy so that they feel more confident to handle difficult situations. Parents should also be aware that the results of this study support the belief that children with food allergies are resilient.

Ultimately, children with food allergies need to accept their food allergy as a part of their life, and not be consumed by it. An important goal would be to help children develop an age-appropriate, sense of control over their food allergies so that their self-confidence begins to build at an early age. This will require continued efforts by you to support and monitor how well your child is able to manage his/her food allergy. For youngsters, both too little control and too much control are problematic, so it is important to strive for a healthy balance.

In order to accomplish this goal, it is critical that even when children are quite young, they are made aware of their food allergy and understand in an age-appropriate way, what this will mean for them. To help them begin to do this, it is recommend that you set up three simple "rules for safety" which should remain steadfast for the toddler and preschooler: **1.)** a food may be eaten only after seeking *your* approval, **2.)** a food should never be shared, and **3.)** you should be told right away if he or she is not feeling well. It is important for children with food allergies to understand that they have a role in helping to keep safe, and in this way, you are helping them to have age-appropriate and reasonable control of their food allergies.

As they get a little older, set up safe parameters in their environment outside of the house. For children who will attend preschool, teach them who the "go to" person is if they have a question or problem. Let your child know exactly what foods you have approved as safe to eat. Teach your child that it is o.k. to say "no" if a food is offered which you did not explicitly indicate was safe. Teach your child how important it is to let the "go to" person know right away if he or she isn't feeling well. Role playing different scenarios is a wonderful way to help children get more comfortable with speaking up for themselves, especially for those children for whom this does not come easily. By including food-allergic children in the plan for their safety, you are helping them to learn and incorporate practical skills they will need in order to keep themselves safe. You are also helping them to begin the process of believing in themselves and their ability to care for themselves. This builds self-confidence and will help them to develop a positive self-concept.

As your child enters elementary school, your efforts to keep your child safe will continue. At this time, more opportunities for higher risk situations will present themselves, as will your child's desire and need for more independence. His/her friendship circle may grow. School-aged children's awareness of social engagements will also grow as may their desire to participate in these events. This scenario will undoubtedly cause a very real conflict of opposing emotions within you: "Do I let my child participate, or do I keep him or her home where I know it is safe?" As discussed earlier, adopting a practical approach to evaluate the pros and cons of the situation in question is always helpful. Consider your child's feelings as part of your criteria as you decide whether or not to allow him or her to participate in the activity. It is important to reconcile this conflict and work it out so that your child may continue to move through the childhood developmental stages of independence and autonomy. Part of this process means that your role will become more "behind the scenes" as you work to gather information regarding school curriculum and events. It is also important that your child continues to be involved in helping to manage his/her food allergies, again, in an age appropriate way. Talk to your child about the plan, and *what his/her role is* in that plan. Advance planning is key and will help to reduce "surprises". This will serve to reduce stress for both you and your child.

Continue to guide your child as you begin the process of "passing the baton" to him or her. Children with food allergies must be taught important life-skills they will need to manage their food allergies, such as always having their medicine with them, not eating food unless they have carefully checked for safe ingredients, having safe foods available when appropriate, knowing when to speak up and ask questions, washing their hands before and after eating, understanding how to use their EpiPen® as they get older, training their friends in how to administer the EpiPen®, and always having a cell phone in case of an emergency. Role play and talk about such things as when it is o.k. to say yes to food, and how your child might say no to a food or situation that feels unsafe.

For parents of teenagers with a food allergy, having patience and a sense of humor will go a long way towards making life easier. It is important to try and have faith in what your child has learned and to trust in his/her ability to do the things necessary to stay safe. Be sensitive to the many emotions your child may experience. Your child needs to know that his/her feelings and opinions are important to you. This is a critical time to work hard at keeping the lines of communication open between you and your teenager. Listen to your child when he or she expresses thoughts and feelings to you and make yourself available to offer your support, understanding and advice, when needed.

Teenagers must learn to advocate for themselves with both peers and adults. This is not always an easy proposition. Developing and maintaining a positive attitude can go a long way in making difficult situations better. Children, and especially young adults, need to feel that they can control their food allergies, rather than feel that their food allergies are controlling them. Encourage your child to adopt a practical approach to managing his/her food allergies and focus on what *can* be done and not what can't be done. The goal for parents is to help their children with food allergies develop the skills to become confident and creative problem-solvers so that they can keep ***moving forward***.

Helen Keller expressed a philosophy about life from which we could all benefit. She said, "Life is about change. We can only find true happiness when we move forward and embrace the experience."

A CAREFUL, CONFIDENT APPROACH

The resilience of children with food allergies and their families is truly impressive. But it's important for families to understand that they are not alone in experiencing emotional responses to life with food allergy, and that these responses will likely ebb and flow in the context of children's development and life events. At times, children can experience feelings of sadness, anger, and frustration related to restrictions on foods and activities, or self-consciousness about standing out from peers due to their allergies. Parents, too, can feel isolated and frustrated when it seems family and friends "just don't get it." New diagnoses, allergic reactions, and developmental milestones associated with less direct parental supervision, such as entering school, can all be associated with anxiety for parents and children, as can children's greater understanding of risks as they get older, and even the unknown of what it would be like to have a serious reaction or receive emergency medication. The important thing is that when parents model a careful, but confident approach to allergy management, involve children in planning ways to participate in activities, and provide positive attention for children's coping efforts, children can benefit from the underlying message that food allergy is manageable, and that they are not defined by their allergies.

Jennifer LeBovidge, Ph.D.
Psychologist, Children's Hospital, Boston, Massachusetts

For School Personnel

This chapter presents a comprehensive overview of the psychological distress which may be experienced by children diagnosed with food allergy, and the wide range of emotional responses possible to this health condition. Efforts made by the student to avoid food allergens may be a catalyst for anxiety and worry, exclusion from social activities may cause feelings of sadness and frustration, and teasing or bullying from peers will undoubtedly create a myriad of emotions from fear to anger to shame. Studies clearly demonstrate that a diagnosis of food allergy negatively impacts quality of life issues for these individuals. School personnel, in addition to addressing the physical safety of their food-allergic students, play an important role in facilitating the emotional health of these children in regards to their social development.

Following are recommendations to offer guidance to educators in their efforts to address the emotional needs of their students with food allergy:

- Be familiar with the signs of psychosocial distress, as discussed earlier in this chapter, which might be exhibited by a student with food allergy. Have systems in place which facilitate the student's access to assistance, when necessary, such as formal or informal meetings with the teacher, the school nurse, or the school adjustment counselor. It is always extremely helpful for at least one school staff member to develop a comfortable, working relationship with the student, and typically that person is the school nurse or the teacher.

- Classroom plans should be designed which enable the food-allergic student to participate safely, along with his/her peers, in the academic program as well as in extra-curricular and social activities. This inevitably requires advance planning and a multi-disciplinary approach to be adopted by the teacher, the school nurse, and the principal, for example. The student's parents should be regarded as part of the team and be utilized as a resource whenever questions arise about the safety of foods and/or materials. The rule of thumb should be that all students within the class should benefit equally from the curriculum offered. In the elementary grades, well thought-out safe snack programs and birthday/holiday celebrations are necessary for a safe physical environment. This approach will also allow children with food allergies to relax and fully enjoy the social aspects implicit in these activities.

- For lunch in the cafeteria, arrangements should be implemented which insure that other children with safe lunches will sit at the table with the food-allergic student. Again, this reassures the child with food allergies that he or she is physically safe, while also allowing for important social interaction and development.

- Make sure the student with food allergies 1.) understands the procedures to be implemented in the plan for his/her safety, and 2.) understands his/her role in that plan.

- Utilize the opportunity to develop lesson plans which explain the health condition of food allergy and promote discussions about our differences. These activities can have a profound effect on peer acceptance and tolerance of food allergy-related practices in the classroom, which in turn, will have a positive effect on the food-allergic student's sense of comfort in the school environment. Lesson plans of this nature can easily be incorporated into the Health Curriculum Framework.

- Accept a zero tolerance for bullying or harassment. Have written policies in place that make it clear that such incidents will not be tolerated.

Conclusion

It is important to understand that having a food allergy is more than just a physical issue: the focus must be on the whole child. The health condition of food allergy will clearly have implications on the emotional health of the allergic child and his/her family. Achieving a healthy balance between keeping the child physically safe, while also allowing for the development of "normal" life experiences, is essential to overall well-being. Allowing for experiences which keep children with food allergies safe, but which also allow them to thrive socially and emotionally, will aid them in building a foundation to deal successfully with the lifelong challenges having a food allergy presents.

Help the child with food allergies, in an age-appropriate way, discover how *he or she* can deal effectively with the realities of food allergy on a daily basis. These children need to feel confident in their ability to keep safe and make good decisions. They also need to know that they can have fun and enjoy life. If children with food allergies are successful in adopting an attitude of positive perseverance, despite obstacles that might stand in their way, their chances of having a better quality of life will be greatly enhanced. You will have achieved a great accomplishment if you are able to encourage and help the child with food allergies develop this attitude and approach towards life.

KNOWLEDGE + SUPPORT = SUCCESS

"The test of success is not what you do when you are on top.
Success is how high you bounce when you hit the bottom."
General George S. Patton

"I attribute my success to this: I never gave or took an excuse."

Florence Nightingale

CHAPTER SIX

ANALYSIS OF A SCHOOL NURSE SURVEY ON FOOD ALLERGY MANAGEMENT

BACKGROUND

Research indicates that food allergy affects 3 million school-aged children (ages 5-18) in the United States. The impact this statistic has on schools is made clear when we consider that one in every five children with a food allergy will experience an allergic reaction at school. Furthermore, 40-50% of individuals diagnosed with a food allergy are considered to have a high risk of experiencing a life-threatening reaction, or anaphylaxis. Add to this the fact that food allergens are responsible for 30% of fatal anaphylaxis, and the connection between food allergies and schools becomes particularly profound.

Several studies conducted over the past ten years have investigated how food allergies are managed at school. A study entitled, "Food-allergic Reactions in Schools and Preschools," published in the *Archives of Pediatric and Adolescent Medicine* in 2001, found that it is common for children to experience an allergic reaction to food at school. Despite this likelihood, however, only 67% of the eighty schools participating in this study made at least one accommodation to reduce the risk of allergen exposure for their food-allergic students. Also noteworthy is the fact that 16% of the students in this study who experienced a food-induced allergic reaction at school, did not have medication available for treatment. Another study published in 2000 in the *Journal of Allergy and Clinical Immunology,* "Allergic Reactions to Foods in School", sought to determine the characteristics of allergic reactions experienced at school. Variability was found regarding the location where medications used to treat allergic reactions were maintained at school. Medications were kept with the school nurse in the Health Office—46%, with the student's teacher—23%, in the student's bag—18%, and in the school's front office—15%. In addition, 9% of the elementary school children in this study did not have a treatment plan or medications available at the time of their allergic event.

A more recent study entitled: "Impact of Food Allergies on School Nursing Practice" was published in the *Journal of School Nursing* in October, 2004. This nation-wide telephone survey of 400 elementary school nurses evaluated the ways in which food allergies are managed by school nurses. This study found that:

- 44% of the nurses reported an increase in the number of children with food allergies over the last 5 years, and that peanuts were the most common food allergen,

- only 78% of the nurses did staff training as a preventive strategy, and

- 90% of the nurses kept epinephrine primarily in their office.

This study drew the following conclusions:

- school staff were not adequately prepared to effectively manage food allergies at school, and consequently, more consistent training for school staff needs to occur,

- epinephrine needs to be stored in a location that allows for timely access for its administration, and,

- epinephrine should be stored in a safe location, but never in a locked cabinet during the school day.

An important article which offers guidance and information on this subject written by Michael C. Young, MD, Ann Munoz-Furlong, BA and Scott H. Sicherer, MD, was published in the August, 2009, *Journal of Allergy and Clinical Immunology*. The authors reviewed numerous studies on school food allergy management and highlighted two main deficiencies:

1.) the inadequate establishment and implementation of food allergy management plans, and

2.) the inadequate recognition of symptoms of anaphylaxis and treatment with epinephrine.

This article stresses the need for schools to develop policies for food allergy management which include both a <u>plan for the avoidance of food allergens</u> and a <u>plan for the treatment of allergic reactions and anaphylaxis</u>.

An annual report written by the Massachusetts Department of Public Health (MA DPH) on the epidemiology of epinephrine administrations for the treatment of life threatening allergic reactions in public and private schools in Massachusetts offers additional information of relevance to this topic. The report for the school year 2008-2009, found that for 131 reporting schools, there were 175 administrations of epinephrine by auto-injector (154 for students, 13 for adult staff, 3 for visitors and for 5 the status was unknown). Symptoms of allergic reactions developed in locations throughout the school environment, including in the classroom—39%, in the cafeteria—14%, in the health office—15%, on the playground—6%, and in the gym—4%. Additional information of interest:

- Food was responsible for the majority of anaphylactic reactions (42%), the cause was unknown in 33% of reactions, insect sting and "other" (medication, latex, etc.) were responsible for the remaining 25% of reactions.

- The most frequently reported allergies were to peanuts and nuts.

- 38 individuals (22%) were not known to have an allergic condition at the time of their anaphylactic event.

- In 89% of cases, epinephrine was administered by the school nurse.

- Only 76% of individuals with a known allergy had an individual healthcare plan in place at the time of their anaphylactic event.

PURPOSE AND GOAL

"School Nurse Survey on Food Allergy Management"

Four facts regarding food allergies are clear: 1.) the number of school-aged children developing food allergies is growing, with no sign of abating, 2.) a significant number of students are experiencing allergic reactions and anaphylaxis at school which require treatment with epinephrine, making the school setting a high risk environment for these students, 3.) schools have a responsibility to address the safety needs of their students with food allergies, and 4.) school nurses are the key players in this effort, and are faced with the challenging task of minimizing the risk of food-allergen exposure for their students, and being prepared to treat a reaction, should one occur.

The purpose of this school nurse survey was to determine the strategies utilized by school nurses in Massachusetts to manage their students' food allergies. Questions on the survey were designed to investigate procedures utilized by the school nurses for the prevention and treatment of food-induced anaphylaxis. Analysis of the nurses' responses to the survey provides important information for school personnel and families as they work to find field-tested, practical and effective strategies for the management of this health condition within the school environment. Ultimately, the goal of this survey is to:

1.) facilitate a better understanding of current food allergy management practices,

2.) highlight reasonable strategies utilized which are meant to enhance the safety of food-allergic students at school and allow them to be fully engaged in their school programs, including both academic and extra-curricular activities, and

3.) solicit from practicing school nurses their opinions regarding the most important factors which either promote or detract from school food allergy management efforts.

Nurses were asked to comment on what they believe is the most important procedure to implement at school in order to help prevent a student from having an allergic reaction, what they have found to be the most difficult aspect of managing a student with food allergies, and what they have found to be the most helpful aspect of making their program work best. The nurses' responses will allow important insights to be drawn regarding factors which they perceive may foster or inhibit the success of their efforts to implement risk reduction and treatment procedures. To date, this may be the first survey designed to solicit this type of information.

METHOD

A fifty-question survey was developed by the private consulting company, Educating For Food Allergies, LLC (EFFA), to ascertain school food allergy management practices currently being utilized in school settings. The subjects were sixty-nine (69) pre-school, elementary, middle and high school nurses who represented public, charter and private schools located throughout all regions of Massachusetts. These 69 nurses attended a professional development workshop offered by EFFA on school food allergy management: forty-seven (47) elementary school nurses, ten (10) middle school nurses, six (6) high school nurses, four (4) elementary/middle school nurses, and two (2) pre-school nurses. These nurses attended one of several dates offered for this workshop, over the time period of the academic school years 2008-2009, and 2009-2010. Surveys were distributed before the workshop began, as the nurses arrived, and were collected at the end of the program. Surveys were completed anonymously, with the exception of indicating the school level in which each nurse was assigned. Because this survey was designed as a self-report questionnaire, not all questions on every survey were answered.

RESULTS

The number of students with a documented food allergy reported by school nurses in their building ranged from as few as two to as many as seventy. The average number of students with a documented food allergy per building was eighteen.

District Policy

Thirty-three school nurses (48%) reported that their school district has a life threatening allergy (LTA) policy in writing. Seventeen nurses (25%) did not answer this question, which would most likely indicate that there is no LTA policy in their district, or that they are not aware of the existence of a district LTA policy, which is problematic in either case.

Plans for Treatment

EpiPen® Administration Training

Training on EpiPen® administration was conducted for *all* school staff by forty-seven nurses (68%). Twenty-two nurses (32%) conducted EpiPen® administration training for *only* staff who would be given the responsibility of treating a student should they experience anaphylaxis.

Epinephrine

Not every student with a food allergy provided an EpiPen® to the school nurse. Thirty nurses (43.4%) reported that they had fewer EpiPen®s than students with a documented food allergy at school. Thirty-eight nurses (55%) recommended that each food-allergic student provide the nurse with more than one EpiPen®.

Twenty-two nurses (32%) surveyed kept the EpiPen®s only with them in the Health Room, and in no other location within the school environment. Seventeen nurses (25%) surveyed kept EpiPen®s in both the Health Room and in the student's classroom, and four of these nurses reported having a procedure for the classroom teacher to pass off a fanny pack containing the EpiPen®, to the Specialist (art, music, etc.). The Specialist would then return the fanny pack to the classroom teacher at the termination of class. Three of the four nurses who utilized this procedure found it to be effective, whereas the fourth nurse reported it to be ineffective because the teacher often forgot to bring the medicine when leaving the classroom. This specific procedure was only reported at the elementary school level. Twelve nurses (17%) kept EpiPen®s in stationary locations in addition to the Health Room, including in the student's classroom, cafeteria, gym, principal's office, and main office.

Eighteen out of sixty-nine nurses (26%) surveyed had a procedure for the food-allergic student to carry his/her own EpiPen®, most often in a fanny pack, backpack or purse. The ages of students given this responsibility ranged from six to eighteen. Only eight out of forty-seven (17%) of the elementary school nurses had their food-allergic students carry their own EpiPen®. Statistically, the practice of having the students carry their own EpiPen® was reported most often at the middle and high school levels.

Thirty-four nurses (49%) responded that there is an EpiPen®-trained staff member present for before/after school-sponsored events.

Anaphylaxis at School

Fifteen out of sixty-nine nurses (22%) reported that they treated a student with epinephrine for anaphylaxis experienced at school. Peanuts or nuts were known to be responsible for seven cases (47%), cantaloupe was responsible for one case, and in the remaining cases, the food responsible was listed as "unknown" or was simply not listed. Thirteen out of the fifteen cases (87%) involved an elementary school student, and two out of the fifteen cases (13%) involved a middle school student. In fourteen out of the fifteen cases, (93%), it was the school nurse who administered the EpiPen®. In one case of anaphylaxis, the parent administered the EpiPen® to her child with the school nurse's supervision. In two out of fifteen cases of anaphylaxis (13%), a second dose of epinephrine was required, and in both cases, it was administered by the responding EMTs. Two nurses who administered epinephrine for anaphylaxis reported that not all students with a food allergy have a written emergency treatment plan (ETP) in place at school (13%). Three of the students (21%) who experienced anaphylaxis at school were not reported to have an Individual Healthcare Plan (IHP) in place at the time of their anaphylactic event.

School nurses who treated a student for anaphylaxis reported seeing the following symptoms: facial swelling, flushed skin, hives, swelling of the lips and tongue, itchy mouth and throat, eczema flare, lung congestion, difficulty breathing, coughing and wheezing. Not all anaphylactic reactions were reported to include hives. Nurses also reported that students in two instances said they "felt funny" and "did not feel well".

Nurses reported the following foods as allergenic for their students:

Most prevalent—peanuts, tree nuts (walnuts, pecans, pine nuts), milk, egg, soy, shellfish, wheat, sesame seeds.

Less prevalent—apples, beans, beef, carrots, kiwi, corn, peas, strawberries, turkey, chicken, pork, pineapple, chocolate, coconut, peach, lamb, peppers, cantaloupe, raspberries, lime, lemon, avocado, potato, oats, barley, tahini, mustard, cottonseed, banana, sunflower seeds, poppy seeds, blueberries, chick peas, tuna.

Five nurses also reported having students with a latex allergy.

Emergency Treatment Plan (ETP)

Fifty-five out of a total of sixty-nine nurses (78%) reported that all students with a food allergy in their building have a written emergency treatment plan in place at school. For elementary school nurses, 83% reported having ETPs in place for all food-allergic students, for middle school nurses, 66% reported all students with food allergies had an ETP, for high school nurses, 80% reported their food-allergic students had an ETP, and 100% of the preschool nurses reported ETPS were in place for their students with food allergies. Thirteen out of fifteen nurses (87%) who treated a student for anaphylaxis reported that all food-allergic students had a written treatment plan in place at their school. Two out of fifteen nurses (13%) who treated a student with anaphylaxis reported that not all students had a treatment plan in place in their school.

Plans for Prevention/Risk Reduction

Education—General Food Allergy Training

Forty-eight nurses (69%) said that they conduct a general training on food allergies to *all* school staff.

Individual Healthcare Plans

Fifty-five out of sixty-nine nurses (80%) reported managing their students' food allergies proactively with an Individual Healthcare Plan (IHP), a 504 Plan, or a 504 Plan with an IHP attached. Specifically, forty-one out of sixty-nine school nurses (59%) reported managing their food-allergic students with only Individual Healthcare Plans (IHPs), two out of sixty-nine nurses (3%) reported using only 504 Plans, six out of sixty-nine nurses (8.7%) reported using either an IHP or a 504 Plan, and six out of sixty-nine nurses (8.7%) reported using a 504 Plan with an IHP attached. Fourteen out of sixty-nine nurses (20%) indicated that they did not use any plan for prevention to manage their students' food allergies.

To initiate a plan for prevention for a student with food allergies, whether as an IHP or a 504 Plan, thirty-four out of sixty-nine nurses (49%) responded that school personnel made the initial contact with the family, six out of sixty-nine nurses (8.6%) responded that the parent made the initial contact with the school, and ten out of sixty-nine nurses (14%) indicated it was case-dependent, and that either the school staff or the parent made the initial contact to begin this process.

"Peanut-Free" Designations

School-wide: Only four out of sixty-nine schools (6%) were given a designation of being "peanut-free". Three of these were elementary schools, and one was a preschool.

Classrooms: In answer to the question, "Does your school offer peanut/tree nut free classrooms?", thirty-two out of sixty-nine nurses (46%) responded "Yes". For preschool nurses, one out of two (50%) reported that peanut-free classrooms were available, for elementary school nurses, twenty-three out of forty-seven (49%) reported that peanut-free classrooms were offered, two out of four elementary/middle school nurses (50%) reported peanut-free classrooms were available, four out of ten middle school nurses (40%) reported peanut-free classrooms were available, and two out of six high school nurses (33%) reported peanut-free classrooms were available.

Avoidance of other Food Allergens

In answer to the question, "Does your school offer classrooms that are free of other allergens (e.g. milk, sesame, egg, etc.)?", only nine out of sixty-nine nurses (13%) reported that this accommodation was offered. Eight were elementary school nurses, and one was a middle school nurse. Nurses reported that the following foods were avoided in designated classrooms: milk, soy, mustard, corn, sesame, oats, wheat and barley.

Foods in the Classroom for Snack and Celebrations

Twenty-nine out of sixty-nine nurses (42%) reported that *all* snacks brought in to "allergen-free" classrooms are allergen-free. One nurse out of sixty-nine reported that no snacks at all were allowed in these classrooms. Thirty-eight nurses (55%) reported that their school allows food celebrations in the allergen-free classrooms. Of the thirty-eight nurses who indicated that food is allowed for celebrations, twenty-three (60.5%) reported that all of these foods are allergen-free for the food-allergic student(s). Only thirty-seven out of sixty-nine nurses (54%) reported that it is the responsibility of an adult to check for safe ingredients for snacks brought into the classroom. Comments included: "it is the teacher's responsibility to check", "the parent is notified when food is brought into the classroom", "only store-bought food is allowed", "parents must send in an ingredient list or the food is not allowed", "the students with food allergies only eat food brought from home".

Food used in School-wide Celebrations

For food at school-wide events, sixteen out of sixty-nine nurses (23%) reported that there are procedures to make *all* food at these events peanut/tree nut free. When peanut and nut products are present at school-wide events, thirty-four nurses (49%) reported that there are procedures to facilitate the safe participation of the food-allergic student. It should be noted that approximately one half of the total number of nurses responding to this survey chose not to answer this question.

The Cafeteria

Fifty-one out of sixty-nine nurses (68%) reported that a peanut-free table is available in the cafeteria. A peanut-free table was reported to be provided more often at the elementary school level, thirty-nine out of forty-seven (83%), as opposed to its availability at the middle or high school level, eight out of sixteen (50%). Sixteen out of sixty-nine nurses (23%) report that a table free of other food allergens, in addition to peanuts/nuts, is available in the cafeteria. This practice was more common at the elementary school level.

Forty-one out of sixty-nine nurses (59%) report that an adult staff member is assigned to monitor the allergen-free table. This practice was reported for all school levels. Of the thirty-nine elementary school nurses who report the availability of a peanut-free table in the cafeteria, thirty-two nurses (82%) answered that there is an adult staff member assigned to monitor the table for safe ingredients. Forty-seven out of sixty-nine school nurses (68%) report that there is a plan used to insure that other students with safe lunches also sit at the allergen-free table with the food-allergic student.

Hand Washing

Hand washing practices by the food-allergic student is used as a preventive measure against food-allergen exposure by sixty out of sixty-nine nurses (87%). Thirty-nine nurses (56%) reported using hand washing procedures for *all* students in the food-allergic student's classroom as a preventive measure against allergen exposure. Nurses reported that soap and water and/or wipes are used most often for hand washing practices.

Field Trips

Fifty-eight out of sixty-nine nurses (84%) reported that they do not go on all field trips attended by a food-allergic student. For the fifty-eight nurses who do not go on all field trips, fifty-five (94%) report that an EpiPen®-trained staff member attends the field trip. Fifty-one out of sixty-nine nurses (74%) report that the parent of the food-allergic student is always invited to attend the field trip. Elementary school nurses were more likely to invite the food-allergic student's parent to attend the field trip—thirty-eight out of forty-seven (81%).

Bus Transportation

Only twenty-three out of sixty-nine nurses (33%) reported that school bus drivers are trained in EpiPen® administration. One hundred percent of the forty-six remaining nurses in this survey who reported that bus drivers are not trained in EpiPen® administration, also report that there is not an EpiPen® trained staff member who rides the bus. Noteworthy comments included: "company refuses training", "these students don't ride the bus", "no training is conducted, per bus company policy", "we were conducting training, but the new bus company stopped", "only SPED bus drivers are EpiPen® trained".

Nineteen out of sixty-nine nurses (27.5%) reported that an EpiPen® is readily available on the bus, thirty-three nurses (48%) indicated epinephrine is not readily available on the bus, and seventeen nurses (25%) were unsure. When epinephrine is readily available on the bus, sixteen out of nineteen nurses (84%) reported that it is carried by the student; two nurses (10.5%) report that it is carried by the bus driver; and one nurse (5%) responded that it is carried by the bus monitor. The location of the EpiPen® while on the school bus was reported to be in either a fanny pack, a backpack or in a purse.

Emotional Distress Related to Food Allergy

Nurse participants in this survey were asked if they have worked with food-allergic students who have exhibited signs of stress, anxiety, denial and/or depression which they believed to be associated in full or in part, with having a food allergy. Twenty-six out of sixty-nine nurses (37.6%) reported that they have witnessed signs of stress, thirty-two nurses (46%) reported they have witnessed signs of anxiety, six nurses (8.6%) reported that they have witnessed signs of denial, and three nurses (4%) have witnessed signs of depression.

Factors which Promote School Food Allergy Management

School nurses were asked what they believe is the most important procedure that needs to be implemented at school in order to help prevent a student from having a food-allergic reaction. The most prevalent response was "education", which was offered by twenty-eight out of sixty-nine nurses (40.5%). Education was stated as being important for staff, for parents and for students. The second most prevalent answer was "communication and information sharing", which was received from nine nurses (13%). Additional responses included: hand washing, allergen avoidance, having a formal or written IHP and ETP, no food at parties, allergen-free zones, quick access to medicine, meeting with the food-allergic student's parents, identification of the food-allergic student to school staff, parents acting as an advocate for their child, no food sharing, checking snacks for ingredients, and more staff willing to be EpiPen® trained.

School nurses were asked what they have found to be the most helpful aspect of making their program work best. Answers given most often were: education of staff, staff support and cooperation, administrative support, development of a good relationship with the food-allergic student's parents which "raises confidence and decreases anxiety", close contact with the teachers throughout the school year, communication between all parties (including reminder letters at holiday times), having written plans (IHP, ETP), allergen-safe zones (classroom and in the cafeteria).

Factors which make School Food Allergy Management Difficult

School nurses were asked what they have found to be the most difficult aspect of managing students with a food allergy at school. The two most prevalent answers to this question were 1.) food at classroom parties, and 2.) lack of cooperation from staff and parents of non-allergic students with regards to risk reduction procedures. Additional answers included: difficulty getting cooperation/support from school administration, difficulty getting EpiPen®s, doctor's orders and related information from parents of the food-allergic students, field trips, the cafeteria, anxiety/emotions of parents of food-allergic students, and having responsibility for a large number of students at school with food allergies.

Helpful elements of the Massachusetts Department of Education's (MA DOE) guidelines, "Managing Life Threatening Food Allergies in Schools"

Thirty-two out of sixty-nine school nurses (46%), use the MA DOE guidelines as a resource in their food allergy management planning. School nurses reported that they use the Massachusetts school food allergy management guidelines most often for: education and training of their staff, for assistance in writing care plans for their food-allergic students, and for guidance in policy development. Additional comments included that the guidelines were used for ideas and as a reference for parents, when needed.

In answer to the question, "What have you found most helpful about the MA DOE guidelines?", school nurses reported that the guidelines offer good, concrete information and are clearly written, structured and easy to understand. Additional comments included that the MA DOE's food allergy guidelines were helpful in getting the process started for staff training, policy development, and in providing an explanation of the responsibilities of the nurse, teacher, parent, etc., in relation to school food allergy management.

DISCUSSION

Plans for Treatment

Previous research has demonstrated that food-induced anaphylaxis occurs at school, a fact which is further confirmed by this survey's results. Numerous studies have also indicated that peanuts or nuts are the most common foods responsible for allergic reactions requiring treatment with epinephrine at school, a conclusion which is also consistent with the findings of this survey. The availability of epinephrine to promptly treat severe allergic reactions and anaphylaxis is an obvious and crucial component of any emergency response plan. This appears to present a significant problem for nearly one-half (43.4%) of the Massachusetts school nurses surveyed, however, who reported that they did not receive an EpiPen® for every student in their school diagnosed with a food allergy. Frustration was expressed by many of the nurses who, despite repeated requests, failed to receive this life-saving medicine from the families of all of their food-allergic students. Treatment of a life-threatening allergic reaction for students diagnosed with a food allergy, but who do not provide an EpiPen® to the school, requires that emergency treatment be administered by responding EMTs. This possible scenario raises serious concerns for a positive outcome given the fact that a delay in receiving epinephrine is determined to be a significant risk factor for fatal anaphylaxis. It is possible that the cost of epinephrine auto-injectors may be prohibitive for some families. Nonetheless, education for parents of children with food allergies as to the reasons why they must provide EpiPen®s to the school, becomes an important initiative, if the school is to receive the medication it requires in order to respond appropriately to a student's anaphylactic event.

Keeping epinephrine in a location where it is readily accessible reduces the likelihood that a delay will occur in receiving this life-saving medicine. A generally accepted recommendation is for epinephrine by auto-injector to be kept in several locations throughout the school environment where the food-allergic student is considered to be at most risk. The appropriateness of this recommendation is supported by the 2008-2009 Massachusetts DPH epinephrine administration report which demonstrated that students experienced anaphylaxis not only in the Health Room, but also in the classroom, gym, playground, and cafeteria. Sixty-eight percent of nurses responding to this survey have procedures which address the need for timely access to epinephrine. These procedures include keeping EpiPen®s in their Health Room *and* in other safe locations where the child presumably will be at most risk (the student's classroom, the cafeteria and gym), and/or having arrangements for the EpiPen® to be carried by the student or adult staff as the child moves throughout the school environment. The practice of having staff carry the food-allergic student's medicine was implemented by a relatively small number of elementary school nurses (8.5%), and not by any middle or high school nurses. Plans that allow the food-allergic student to carry the EpiPen® were utilized more often by middle and high school nurses as compared with elementary school nurses in this survey.

Timely access to epinephrine may be a challenge for 32% of the nurses surveyed who reported that they kept students' EpiPen®s in only one location, the Health Room. Nonetheless, this number does represent a significant improvement as compared with the 90% of nurses in the 2004 study referenced earlier ("Impact of food allergy on school nursing practice") who kept their epinephrine auto-injectors primarily in the Health Room.

Before and after school-sponsored events present a high risk for students with food allergies. Only one-half of the nurses surveyed (49%) reported the presence of an EpiPen®-trained staff member during these times. The survey did not ascertain if epinephrine is made available to food-allergic students participating in these activities.

Numerous studies have highlighted the need for *all* students with food allergies to have a written emergency treatment plan (ETP) in place at school. With only 78% of the nurses in this survey reporting that all of their food-allergic students have an ETP, it appears that this is an area that still requires improvement.

Plans for Prevention/Risk Reduction

Avoidance of a student's food allergen is fundamental in reducing the risk of a food-induced allergic reaction. Therefore, general education for school personnel on the signs and symptoms of an allergic reaction and anaphylaxis, and the ways in which a student may be exposed to their allergens, becomes a crucial element of school food allergy management. The more school personnel understand the significance of implementing risk reduction strategies, the less likely are the chances a student with food allergies will experience a severe allergic reaction at school. In addition, when more school staff are able to recognize the symptoms of anaphylaxis, the more likely it becomes that the student experiencing this medical emergency will be treated promptly. Although 69% of the nurses in this survey conduct general training on food allergies to all school personnel, that still leaves almost 31% of the schools where not all staff have been educated on these important concepts.

Avoidance remains the cornerstone of food allergy management plans. The need for individualized, written plans which define procedures for the prevention of allergic reactions for students with food allergies, has been a conclusion of numerous studies and a recommendation made by a multitude of professional organizations and state departments of education. Despite this, 20% of the nurses in the survey reported that they do not manage their food-allergic students with any plan for prevention, including individual healthcare plans (IHPs) or 504 plans. In these instances, food-allergic students do not have the protection necessary to reduce their risk of exposure to food allergens, and are subsequently at a higher risk of having an allergic reaction and/or anaphylaxis at school. Hand and surface washing practices, plans for safe snacks and the implementation of allergen-free zones, are relatively easy procedures to implement, and are critical strategies which enhance the student's safety within the school environment. Food allergy management plans at school which focus solely on a plan for the treatment of an allergic reaction are inadequate in meeting the needs of these students.

Children spend a great deal of the school day in their classrooms, and data has shown that the possibility for a student to experience anaphylaxis in the classroom is significant. As a result, much debate and discussion has occurred between school personnel and parents as to whether peanut-free designations are a risk reduction strategy which should be utilized at school. Although results from this survey indicate that only a small number of schools are designated as "peanut-free" (6%), data indicates that it is much more common for a classroom to be given this designation in elementary school. Twenty-three out of thirty-two nurses (71%) who answered affirmatively that their school offers peanut-free classrooms, were elementary school nurses. Eliminating other food allergens from the classroom is significantly less prevalent, and was reported as an accommodation by only 13% of the nurses, all at the elementary level, with the exception of one middle school.

Confusion seems to exist regarding the definition and subsequent meaning of a classroom's designation as being free of a food allergen. More than one-half of the nurses in this survey (58%) report that not all snacks brought into a classroom which has been assigned as "allergen-free", are free of that allergen. Similarly, only 60.5% of the nurses indicate that all foods brought into these classrooms for holiday/celebrations are "allergen-free". Only one-half of the nurses surveyed (54%) reported that procedures are in place for adult staff to monitor food brought in to these "allergen-free" rooms for safe ingredients.

The presence of allergenic foods in the classroom makes hand washing practices as a preventive measure even more meaningful. A majority of the nurses in the survey (87%) report having procedures in place for their food-allergic students to wash their hands. Only 56% of the nurses, however, implemented hand washing procedures for *all* students in these classrooms, which may increase the likelihood of the food-allergic student's exposure to their allergens through cross-contamination or skin contact when food allergens are permitted.

The cafeteria is another high risk area for students with food allergies who may be exposed to their allergen(s) through ingestion, skin contact, inhalation and cross-contamination. To make matters worse, activities in this environment typically lack the level of control found in the classroom setting. A reasonable risk reduction strategy is to provide a peanut-free table in the cafeteria. A significant number of elementary school nurses in this survey (83%) reported that they utilize this strategy at their school, and have a plan for an adult staff member to monitor activities at the table (82%).

Lunch is a time for children to communicate and interact with their peers in an informal setting. For children with food allergies, it is important that they are afforded this same opportunity for their social development, and are not isolated from their classmates by being seated at the allergen-free table by themselves. Only 68% of the nurses in this survey recognize this need and reported that they have a plan to insure that other students with safe lunches also sit at this table with the food-allergic student.

Because allergic reactions can occur during field trips and while riding the bus to and from school, it is critical that these areas are not overlooked when planning risk reduction strategies. Based on the results of this survey, field trips appear to receive more attention in this regard, than bus transportation. While a majority of school nurses reported that they do not attend field trips (84%), they indicated that in 94% of these cases (fifty-five out of fifty-eight nurses), arrangements are made for an EpiPen®-trained staff member to attend the field trip in their place. Conversely, only a small number of school bus drivers are trained in EpiPen® administration (33%), and in the remaining schools where the bus driver does not have this training (66.6%), nurses reported that without exception, there are no arrangements planned for an EpiPen®-trained adult to ride on the bus. In addition, only a little over one-quarter of the nurses reported that an EpiPen® is readily available on the bus. Data from this survey indicate that bus transportation is a high risk activity for food-allergic students. Serious concerns should be raised as to the safety of food-allergic students who choose to ride the school bus, should they experience anaphylaxis while enroute.

Emotional Distress Related to Food Allergy

Within the school environment, food-allergic students must exercise constant vigilance in their efforts to avoid their allergens, deal with the attitudes, both positive and negative, of individuals within their school community, as well as make efforts towards their academic and extra-curricular achievement. Each of these tasks can be daunting, but collectively, they present a considerable challenge. Not surprising then, is the fact that a significant number of school nurses in this survey reported observing signs of emotional distress (stress, anxiety, denial, depression), in their food-allergic students, which they believed was in some way related to the student's response to having a food allergy. This result is consistent with the findings of previous studies which have investigated quality of life issues of individuals who have chronic health conditions, including food allergy.

A 2001 study entitled, "The impact of childhood food allergy on quality of life" by Scott Sicherer, MD, Sarah Noone, RN, MSN, and Anne Munoz-Furlong, BA, sought to determine the impact of food allergy on the individual diagnosed with this disease, and their family. A children's health questionnaire which had specific questions about food allergy, was mailed to families of children with food allergy. The study concluded that food allergy significantly impacts: 1.) the perception of general health, 2.) the limitation of family activities and 3.) emotional distress in parents. A subsequent study in 2003, "Daily Coping Strategies for Patients and their Families" by Anne Munoz-Furlong, found that the task of managing food allergy affects the life of the student and his/her family on a daily basis. Areas affected include label reading, meal preparation, planning for safe inclusion at school and dealing with the stress which is often a by-product of all of these activities. Additional support for this premise is found in the conclusion of another 2003 study, "Assessment of quality of life in children with peanut allergy" by NJ Avery et al., which determined that quality of life in children with peanut allergy is more negatively impaired as compared with that of children with insulin-dependent diabetes. A more recent study in 2009 by Jennifer LeBovidge, Ph.D, et al., "Assessment of psychological distress among children and adolescents with food allergy", analyzed the scores on standardized measures of psychological distress for sixty-nine children with food allergy, aged eight to seventeen. Results of this study indicate that these children scored the same or lower than normative scores for distress. It is important to note, however, that two areas of significantly higher distress for children with food allergy in this study were found: anxious coping and separation anxiety.

Studies designed to address the subject of food-allergic students' psychosocial response to this health condition are limited in number. Additional research would elicit important information pertaining to the assessment of the emotional impact of food allergy, and in determining coping strategies effective in enhancing the resilience and overall wellbeing of these students. Recommendations based on study findings could be made to school personnel who work with these students with the goal of helping them to thrive and fully benefit from their academic and extra-curricular school activities.

CONCLUSION

State guidelines and school district life threatening allergy (LTA) policies play a vital role in setting standards for the approach a school district takes for food allergy management, and for offering guidance in the development and implementation of protocols and procedures related to this effort. The ultimate success of risk reduction strategies requires a multi-disciplinary approach, and involves the cooperation and support of many individuals in addition to the school nurse, including the principal, teachers, specialists, aides, cafeteria employees, custodial staff, school district administrators, physicians, parents and classmates. School nurses particularly appreciate the support they receive from staff and administrators, and report that this is often the most helpful aspect in making their food allergy management plans work best. Education of the entire school community is necessary so that there is a common understanding of the risks inherent in having a food allergy, of reasonable ways to manage these risks, and how to recognize and treat an allergic reaction. Clear communication of accommodations and procedures to be implemented must be extended to all individuals involved, so that confusion is avoided. This will help to encourage uniform compliance with requests made by teachers to parents of non-allergic students.

Every effort must be employed by the school nurse and the student's parents to insure that *every* student with a diagnosed food allergy has at least one prescribed EpiPen® and an emergency treatment plan (ETP), at school. Written individual healthcare plans (IHPs) must also be developed for *every* student with a food allergy, and these plans should include procedures to reduce the risk of allergen exposure in all areas of the school environment. Two areas highlighted in this survey which pose a particular risk for the safety of students with food allergies and cause considerable concern for many school nurses involve: 1.) food brought into the classroom and 2.) the time during which the student travels on the school bus. School personnel must pay particular attention to these issues in order to develop protocols which maximize the food-allergic student's safety. It is not unusual for these students to experience feelings of stress and anxiety related to their health condition. Food allergy management must focus on the whole student, so that a plan is in place which addresses both the student's physical and emotional wellbeing.

This survey confirms that proactive and comprehensive planning that represent a coordinated effort is required to insure that policies, protocols and procedures are in place which respond appropriately to the needs of students with life-threatening food allergies.

SCHOOL NURSE SURVEY ON FOOD ALLERGY MANAGEMENT

(Developed by: Educating For Food Allergies, LLC)
Spring, 2008

School: _____Elementary _____Middle _____High School

1. Total student population at the school _____

2. Number of students with a documented food allergy _____

    2a. Number of students with multiple food allergies (e.g. more than two) _____

3. Number of students with a prescribed EpiPen® _____

4. Do you recommend that students provide the school with more than one EpiPen®?_____

5. Are EpiPen®s kept in other locations in addition to the nurse's office? _____

    In addition to an EpiPen® set-up in the Nurse's office:

    5a. Are EpiPen®s kept in a safe location in the classroom? _____

    5b. Are EpiPen®s kept in various other locations throughout the school? ___

    5c. If yes, which locations are utilized?_____

6. Is the EpiPen® carried *by the student* during the school day?

7. If yes, what are the ages of students who carry their own EpiPen®?

_____

7a. If yes, where do the students keep their EpiPen® when they travel throughout the school?

_____

8. Is the EpiPen® carried by the teacher and passed to specialists/ adult staff as the student travels during the school day?

_____

8b. If yes, has this been an effective procedure? _____

8c. If not, please explain why_____

_____

9. Do teachers/staff members carry a walkie-talkie outside of the classroom when they are responsible for a student with food allergies? _____

10. Are students with food allergies managed with an IHP_____

10a. *OR* with a 504 Plan _____

10b. *OR* with a 504 Plan, and the IHP attached _____

11. Who made the initial contact to start the process for a student's IHP or 504 Plan, the school or the parent?

_____

12. Do all students with food allergies have a written treatment plan (e.g. "ETP") _____

13. Do you conduct a <u>general training</u> on food allergies to *all* school staff? _____

14. Do you conduct a <u>training</u> on EpiPen® administration for **all** staff? _____

    14a. **OR** Do you conduct EpiPen® administration training **only** for those staff who will be responsible for students with food allergies?_____

15. Is your school registered with the Massachusetts DPH to allow unlicensed staff to be trained to administer the EpiPen®? _____

16. Have you had to use EpiPen® to treat a student with food-induced anaphylaxis? _____

    16a. Have you had to use an EpiPen® to treat **the same student** for food-induced anaphylaxis **for more than one event**? _____

    16b. Briefly, describe the circumstances of each student's allergic reaction.

    _____

    _____

    _____

17. Which staff member gave the student the EpiPen® (for each student, if more than one)?

_____

    17a. Have any students required a second EpiPen®?

    _____

    17b. If yes, which staff member administered the second EpiPen®, **OR** was it administered by EMTs or ER staff? _____

18. Please list all food responsible for food-induced anaphylaxis at your school. _____

_____

19. If your school has a food allergy policy, which terminology is utilized to describe this policy:

   a. "Peanut free" _____

   b. "Peanut/tree nut free" _____

   c. "Peanut/tree nut safe" _____

   d. "Peanut/tree nut aware" _____

   e. "Peanut/tree nut sensitive" _____

   f. Other _____

20. Is your school designated as a peanut/tree nut free school? _____

21. Does your school offer peanut/tree nut free classrooms? _____

22. Does your school offer classrooms that are free of other allergens (e.g. milk, sesame, egg, etc.) _____

   22a. If yes, please list the other allergens
   _____

23. Are *all* students' snacks brought into these classrooms allergen-free? _____

24. Does an adult check all snacks for safe ingredients? _____

25. Does your school allow food celebrations in the allergen-free classrooms? _____

   25a. If yes, are *all* foods brought into the classroom allergen-free?
   _____

26. Do you utilize hand washing practices as a *preventive measure* against food-allergen exposure for the food-allergic student? _____

    26a. If yes, does the student use: soap/water _____ wipes _____ both _____

27. Do all students in these classrooms wash their hands as a *preventive measure?* _____

    27a. If yes, do they use: soap/water _____ wipes _____ both _____

28. If there is more than one student per grade level with a food allergy, are they placed in the same classroom? _____

29. Does a school nurse go on all field trips attended by a food-allergic student? _____

    29a. If not, does an EpiPen® trained staff member attend these field trips? _____

    29b. Is the parent of the food-allergic student always invited to attend the field trip? _____

    29c. Do you send an EpiPen® trained staff member regardless of whether the parent attends? _____

30. Does your school offer a peanut/tree nut free table(s) in the cafeteria? _____

31. Does your school offer tables that are free of other allergens in the cafeteria? _____

32. Is a designated adult assigned to monitor the allergen-free table? _____

33. Is there a plan to insure that other students with peanut/tree nut free lunches will also sit at this table? (e.g. food-allergic student not sitting alone) _____

34. As an alternative, does your school offer designated "peanut/tree nut" tables in the cafeteria? _____

35. Are there procedures to make **all** food at school-wide events peanut/tree nut free? _____

36. If not, are there procedures to facilitate the safe participation of the food-allergic student? _____

37. Do you have EpiPen® trained staff present for before/after school events? _____

38. Are school bus drivers trained in EpiPen® administration? _____

    38a. If no, is there an EpiPen® trained adult on the bus? _____

39. Is EpiPen® readily available on the school bus? _____

    39a. If yes, who carries the EpiPen® on the school bus? _____

40. If yes, where is the EpiPen® kept while on the school bus?
_____

41. Have you worked with food-allergic students who have exhibited signs of:

    a. Stress_____

    b. Anxiety_____

    c. Denial_____

    d. Depression_____

which you believe to be associated in full or in part with having a food allergy?

42. Does your school have a food allergy management policy in writing? _____

43. Does your school *district* have a food allergy management policy in writing? _____

44. What do you believe is the most important procedure that needs to be implemented at school in order to help prevent a student from having a food-allergic reaction?

_____

_____

_____

45. What have you found to be the most difficult aspect of managing students with a food allergy at school?

_____

_____

46. What have you found to be the most helpful aspect of making your program work?

_____

_____

47. In regards to managing students' food allergies at school, how would you describe your relationship with the:

    a. Teacher_____

_____

    b. Parent_____

_____

c. Prinicpal _____

_____

d. Parents of non-allergic students _____

_____

48. Have you used the Massachusetts DOE Food Allergy Management Guidelines as a resource in your planning?_____

48a. If yes, how did you use them?

_____

_____

49. What have you found most helpful about them?

_____

_____

_____

50. What, if anything, would you recommend to improve them?

_____

_____

Copyright© 2008 Educating For Food Allergies, LLC

GLOSSARY

DEFINITION OF TERMS

Anaphylaxis—is a serious allergic reaction that is rapid in onset and may cause death. Fatal reactions may occur without skin symptoms, such as hives, and any food can be the cause of anaphylaxis. Anaphylaxis presents a life-threatening situation and immediate medical treatment is required.

Antihistamine—a drug that blocks the effects of histamine (a chemical released during an allergic reaction), and can be effective in treating symptoms such as itching and hives during a mild allergic reaction. Primarily used for the treatment of hayfever.

Atopic Dermatis—medical term for allergic "eczema".

Basophils—are cells found in the blood. When IgE antibodies attach to them during an allergic reaction, they release chemicals such as histamines that, in turn, cause the symptoms of an allergic reaction.

CAP-RAST and RAST test—are blood tests used to measure the amount of IgE antibodies your body makes to a specific food.

Eczema—refers to a skin condition characterized by red, dry, itchy patches.

Emergency Treatment Plan (ETP)—is the written treatment plan for an individual student, developed by the student's physician/allergist and parent which clearly outlines the steps to follow in the event of an allergic reaction. It should be signed by the physician, the school nurse and the parents.

Epinephrine—the medication that is the treatment of choice to reverse the symptoms of anaphylaxis. It is critical that epinephrine be administered *immediately* if anaphylaxis is suspected. *Epinephrine is a hormone which also occurs naturally in our bodies, known as adrenalin.*

Epinephrine auto-injector—is a spring-based device designed for people without medical training to deliver epinephrine to treat anaphylaxis. Epinephrine auto injectors are sold under the brand names:

- EpiPen® and EpiPen® Jr. auto-injectors—made by Dey Laboratories. Epinephrine is delivered in a single dose, and is available in two doses (EpiPen®—0.3 mg and EpiPen® Jr.—.15 mg). It is sold as a twin-pack.

- Twinject® auto injector—made by Shionogi Pharma, Inc. (previously Verus Pharmaceuticals, Inc.). Delivers one dose of epinephrine, plus has a back-up dose built into the same device.

- Adrenaclick® auto-injector—manufactured by Shionogi Pharma, Inc. Epinephrine is delivered in a single dose, and is available in two doses (0.3 mg and .15 mg). It is available as a single unit or in a twin-pack.

- Generic auto-injector—made by Greenstone® for Shionogi Pharma.

Food Allergic Reaction—is triggered by IgE antibodies to specific food protein, causing release of histamine and other chemical mediators. When this happens, one or several body systems may become involved, such as the skin (rash, swelling), respiratory (sneezing, coughing, difficulty breathing), gastrointestinal (vomiting, diarrhea, abdominal cramps) and cardiovascular (lightheaded, drop in blood pressure), producing the symptoms of an allergic reaction.

Food Allergy—is an abnormal response of the body's immune system to specific food proteins, resulting in allergic reactions with re-exposure to the food.

Hives—raised red areas of the skin that are very itchy, and are usually associated with an allergic reaction.

Histamine—is a chemical released by mast cells and basophils during an allergic reaction that causes allergic symptoms such as itching, hives, swelling, runny nose, wheezing and anaphylaxis.

IgE Antibody—is a food-specific protein found in the blood, and is produced by the body. IgE antibodies attach to mast cells and basophils found in the tissue and blood. This action causes chemicals, such as histamines, to be released, resulting in the symptoms of an allergic reaction. IgE antibodies are detected by CAP RAST tests and skin tests.

Individual Healthcare Plan (IHP)—is a comprehensive, written healthcare plan for an individual student, developed by the school nurse, parents (and student where appropriate) that outlines procedures to be implemented at school intended to reduce the risk of the student from being exposed to an offending allergen and consequently having an allergic reaction.

Mast Cells—are found in body tissues, such as in the nose, throat, lungs, skin, stomach and intestines. When IgE antibodies attach to mast cells during an allergic reaction, it causes the mast cells to release chemicals such as histamines, which in turn, cause the symptoms of an allergic reaction.

<u>Skin Tests</u>—used in allergy testing. In testing for a food allergy, a small prick is made on the skin and a small amount of food extract is put just under the surface of the skin. If a person is allergic to the food being tested, a hive will develop at the site.

<u>The "Big Eight"</u>—refers to the eight foods most likely to cause an allergic reaction; they are: peanuts, tree nuts, wheat, soy, milk, eggs, fish and shellfish.

<u>Urticaria</u>—medical term for hives.

REFERENCES

American Academy of Allergy, Asthma and Immunology. Position Statement: Anaphylaxis in Schools and child-care settings. *J Allergy Clin Immunol* 1998; 102 (2): 173-175.

American Academy of Pediatrics (AAP) Committee on Nutrition (section on Allergy and Immunology)

An Act Concerning Food Allergies and the Prevention of Life-Threatening Incidents. Connecticut Public Act 05-104. 7 June 2005.

An Act Concerning The Administration Of Epinephrine For Certain Students. New Jersey Pub. L. 2007, c. 57. 16 March 2007.

An Act Relating to Education—Health and Safety of Pupils. Rhode Island Pub. L. c. 08-086. 26 June 2008.

Avery NJ, King RM, Knight S, Hourihane JO. "Assessment of quality of life in children with peanut allergy." *Pediatr Allergy Immunol* 2003; 14: 378-82.

Barber, Marianne S. *The Parent's Guide to Food Allergies*. Henry Holt and Company, LLC. New York 2001.

Bock SA, Munoz-Furlong A, Sampson HA. "Further fatalities caused by anaphylactic reactions to food, 2001-6". Letter to editor. *J Allergy Clin Immunol* 2007; 119: 1016-18.

Bock SA, et al. "Fatalities due to anaphylactic reactions to foods." *J Allergy Clin Immunol* 2001; 107: 191-3.

Boyano-Martinez T, et al. "Accidental allergic reactions in children allergic to cow's milk protein." *J Allergy Clin Immunol* 2009; 123: 883-8.

Bryce, JA, et al. Guidelines for the diagnosis and management of food allergy in the United States: Report of the NIAID-sponsored expert panel. *J Allergy Clin Immunol* 2010; 126: S1-S58.

Collins, Lisa Cipriano, M.A., M.F.T. *Caring for Your Child with Severe Food Allergies*. John Wiley & Sons, Inc. New York: 2000.

DunnGalvin A, Gaffney A, Hourihane JO. "Developmental pathways in food allergy: A new theoretical framework." *Allergy* 2009; 64: 560-568.

Erikson, Erik H. *Childhood and Society, 2nd Edition*. W.W. Norton & Company, Inc. New York 1963.

FDA Food Safety Modernization Act, Pub. L. 111-353, § 112 Food Allergy and Anaphylaxis Management, 124 Stat. 3885 (2012).

Fleisher DM, Conover-Walker MK, Christie L, Burks AW, Wood RA. "The natural progression of peanut allergy: Resolution and the possibility of recurrence." *J Allergy Clin Immunol* 2003; 112: 183-9.

Fleischer DM, Conover-Walker MK, Matsui EC, Wood RA. "The natural history of tree nut allergy." *J Allergy Clin Immunol* 2005; 116:1087-1093.

Food Allergen Labeling and Consumer Protection Act of 2004 (FALCPA), Pub. L. 108-282, §201, 118 Stat. 905 (2004).

Food Anaphylaxis Task Force of Massachusetts. "Managing Life Threatening Food Allergies in Schools." Malden, MA. 2002. Massachusetts Department of Education. www.doe.mass.edu/cnp.

Fox AT, et al. "Household peanut consumption as a risk factor for the development of peanut allergy." *J Allergy Clin Immunol* 2009; 123: 417-423.

Gupta, RS, et al. "The Prevalence, Severity, and Distribution of Childhood Food Allergy in the United States." *Pediatrics* 2011; 128: e9-e17.

Hannaway, P.J. M.D. *On the Nature of Food Allergy*. Marblehead, MA. Lighthouse Press 2007.

Hefle SL, Furlong TJ, Niemann L, Lemon-Mule H, Sicherer SH, Taylor SL. "Consumer attitudes and risks associated with packaged foods having advisory labeling regarding the presence of peanuts." *J Allergy Clin Immunol* 2007; 120: 171-6.

Herbst, Sharon Tyler. *The Food Lover's Companion*. Barron's Educational Series, Hauppauge, N.Y. Third Edition 2001.

Hill DJ, et al. "Confirmation of the association between high levels of immunoglobulin E food sensitization and eczema in infancy: an international study." *Clin Exp Allergy* 2008; 38: 161-8.

Ho, MHK, et al. "Early clinical predictors of remission of peanut allergy in children." *J Allergy Clin Immunol* 2008; 121:731-6.

Hourihane J, et al. "An evaluation of the sensitivity of subjects with peanut allergy to very low doses of peanut protein: A randomized, double-blind, placebo-controlled food challenge study." *J Allergy Clin Immunol* 1997; 100: 596-600.

Jones SM, Pons L, Roberts JL, Scurlock AM, Perry TT, Kulis M, et al. "Clinical efficacy and immune regulation with peanut oral immunotherapy." *J Allergy Clin Immunol* 2009; 124: 292-300.

Kemp SF, Lockey RF. "Anaphylaxis: A review of causes and mechanisms." *J Allergy Clin Immunol* 2002; 110: 341-8.

Konstantinou GN, et al. "Consumption of heat-treated egg by children allergic or sensitized to egg can affect the natural course of egg allergy: Hypothesis-generating observations." Letter to the editor. *J Allergy Clin Immunol* 2008; 122: 414-15.

Lack G, et al. "Factors associated with the development of peanut allergy in childhood." *N Engl J Med* 2003; 348: 977-85.

Lack G. "Epidemiologic risks for food allergy." *J Allergy Clin Immunol* 2008; 121: 1331-6.

Lebovidge JS, Strauch H, Kalish LA, Schneider LC. "Assessment of psychological distress among children and adolescents with food allergy." *J Allergy Clin Immunol* 2009; 124: 1282-8.

Lieberman P, Nicklas RA, Oppenheimer J, et al. "The diagnosis and management of anaphylaxis practice parameter: 2010 Update". *J Allergy Clin Immunol* 2010; 126: 477-80.

Longo G, Barbi E, Berti I, Meneghetti R, Pittalis A, Ronfani L, et al. "Specific oral tolerance induction in children with very severe cow's milk-induced reactions." *J Allergy Clin Immunol* 2008; 121: 343-7.

Maleki SJ, et al. "The major peanut allergen, Ara h 2, functions as a trypsin inhibitor, and roasting enhances this function." *J Allergy Clin Immunol* 2003; 112: 190-5.

Maloney JM, et al. "Peanut allergen exposure through saliva: Assessment and interventions to reduce exposure." *J Allergy Clin Immunol* 2006; 118: 719-24.

Massachusetts Department of Public Health, Essential School Health Services Program, Data Report 2007-2008 School Year.

McIntyre CL, et al. "Administration of epinephrine for life-threatening allergic reactions for school settings." *Pediatrics* 2005; 116:1134-40.

Munoz-Furlong A. "Daily coping strategies for patients and their families." *Pediatrics* 2003; 111: 1654-1661.

National Association of School Nurses, Inc. Position Statements: "Individual Healthcare Plans (IHPs)" and "School Nursing

Management of Students with Chronic Health Conditions". www. nasn.org.

Nowak-Wegrzyn A, Isenberg H, Wood RA. "Allergic reactions to foods in the school". *J Allergy Clin Immunol* 2000; 105: S182.

Nowak-Wegrzyn A, Conover-Walker MK, Wood RA. "Food-allergic reactions in schools and preschools". *Arch Pedriatr Adolesc* Med 2001; 155:790-5.

Nowak-Wegrzyn A, et al. "Tolerance to extensively heated milk in children with cow's milk allergy." *J Allergy Clin Immunol* 2008; 122: 342-7.

Perry TT, Conover-Walker MK, Pomes A, Chapman MD, Wood RA. "Distribution of peanut allergen in the environment". *J Allergy Clin Immunol* 2004; 113: 973-6.

Pieretti MM, Chung D, Pacenza R, Slotkin T, Sicherer S. "Audit of manufactured products: Use of allergen advisory labels and identification of labeling ambiguities." *J Allergy Clin Immunol* 2009; 124: 337-41.

Resnick ES, Pieretti MM, Maloney J, Noone S, Munoz-Furlong A, Sicherer SH. "Development of a questionnaire to measure quality of life in adolescents with food allergy: the FAQL-teen." *Ann Allergy Asthma Immunol* 2010; 105 (5): 364-68.

Report of the NIH Expert Panel on Food Allergy Research, March 13-14, 2006. (National Institute of Allergy and Infectious Diseases, National Institutes of Health).

Sampson HA, Mendelson L, Rosen JP. "Fatal and near-fatal anaphylactic reactions to food in children and adolescents." *New England Journal of Medicine* 1992; 327:380-4.

Sampson HA, et al. "Second symposium on the definition and management of anaphylaxis: Summary report—second National

Institute of Allergy and Infectious Disease/Food Allergy and Anaphylaxis Network symposium." *J Allergy Clin Immunol* 2006; 117:391-7)

Savage JH, Matsui EC, Skripak JM, Wood RA. "The natural history of egg allergy." *J Allergy Clin Immunol* 2007; 120: 1413-7.

Savage JH, Kaeding AJ, Matsui EC, Wood RA. "The natural history of soy allergy." *J Allergy Clin Immunol* 2010; 125: 683-6.

School Access to Emergency Epinephrine Act, S.1884, 112th Cong. (2012).

Sicherer SH, et al. "Genetics of peanut allergy: A twin study". *J Allergy Clin Immunol* 2000; 106: 53-6.

Sicherer SH, Noone SA, Munoz-Furlong A. "The impact of childhood food allergy on quality of life." *Ann Allergy Asthma Immunol* 2001; 87:461-464.

Sicherer SH, Munoz-Furlong A, Sampson HA. "Prevalence of peanut and tree nut allergy in the United States determined by means of a random digit dial telephone survey: A 5-year follow-up study". *J Allergy Clin Imunol* 2003; 112:1203-7.

Sicherer SH, Munoz-Furlon A, Sampson HA. "Prevalence of seafood allergy in the United States determined by a random telephone survey". *J Allergy Clin Immunol* 2004; 114: 159-65.

Sicherer,S.H.,M.D. *Understanding and Managing Your Child's Food Allergies*. Baltimore, Maryland. The Johns Hopkins University Press 2006.

Sicherer SH, Simons FER, and the Section on Allergy and Immunology. "Self Injectable Epinephrine for First-Aid Management of Anaphylaxis." *Pediatrics* 2007; 119: 638-646. (AAP Policy).

Sicherer SH. "Peanut allergy: Emerging concepts and approaches for an apparent epidemic." *J Allergy Clin Immunol* 2007; 120: 491-503.

Sicherer SH, Burks AW. "Maternal and infants diets for prevention of allergic diseases: understanding menu changes in 2008." Editorial. *J Allergy Clin Immunol* 2008; 122: 29-33.

Sicherer SH, Leung DYM. "Advances in allergic skin disease, anaphylaxis, and hypersensitivity reactions to foods, drugs, and insects in 2008." *J Allergy Clin Immunol* 2009; 123: 319-27.

Sicherer SH, Leung DYM. "Advances in allergic skin disease, anaphylaxis, and hypersensitivity reactions to foods, drugs, and insects in 2009." *J Allergy Clin Immunol* 2010; 125: 85-97.

Sicherer SH, Munoz-Furlong A, Godbold JH, Sampson HA. "US prevalence of self-reported peanut, tree nut and sesame allergy: 11 year follow-up". *J Allergy Clin Immunol* 2010; 125: 1322-6.

Simons FER. "First-aid treatment of anaphylaxis to food: Focus on epinephrine." *J Allergy Clin Immunol* 2004; 113:837-44.

Simonte SJ, Ma S, Sicherer SH. "Relevance of casual contact with peanut butter in children with peanut allergy." *J Allergy Clin Immunol* 2003; 112:180-2.

Skolnick HS, et al. "The natural history of peanut allergy." *J Allergy Clin Immunol* 2001; 107: 376-74.

Skripak JM, Matsui E, Mudd K, Wood RA. "The natural history of IgE-mediated cow's milk allergy." *J Allergy Clin Immunol* 2007; 120: 1172-7.

Skripak JM, Nash SD, Rowley H, Brereton NH, Ph S, Hamilton RG, et al. "A randomized, double-blind, placebo-controlled study of milk oral immunotherapy for cow's milk allergy." *J Allergy Clin Immunol* 2008; 122: 1154-60.

Srivastava KD, Qu C, Zhang T, Goldfarb J, Sampson HA, Li X-M. "Food Allergy Herbal Formula-2 silences peanut-induced anaphylaxis for a prolonged posttreatent period via IFN-γ-producing CD8+ T cells." *J Allergy Clin Immunol* 2009; 123: 443-51)

The Allergy and Anaphylaxis Management Act of 2007. New York Pub. Health L. § 2500-h. 3 Jan 2007.

The School Nurse's Source Book of Individualized Healthcare Plans, Volume 2, Arnold, Martha J. and Silkworth, Cynthia K., Editors, Sunrise River Press, North Branch, MN, 1999.

United States Department of Agriculture, Food and Nutrition Service. "Accommodating Children with Special Dietary Needs in the School Program. Guidance for School Food Service Staff". Washington, D.C, Fall, 2001.

Weiss C, Munoz-Furlong A, Furlong TJ, Arbit J. "Impact of Food Allergies on School Nursing Practice". *The Journal of School Nursing* 2004; 20: 268-278.

Young MC. "Common Beliefs About Peanut Allergies: Fact or Fiction?" *Food Allergy and Anaphylaxis Network Newsletter*, June-July 2003, p. 9.

Young, M.C., M.D. *The Peanut Allergy Answer Book, 2nd Edition.* Gloucester, MA. Fair Winds Press 2006.

Young MC, Munoz-Furlong A, Sicherer SH. "Management of food allergies in schools: A perspective for allergists." *J Allergy Clin Immunol* 2009;124:175-182.

REFERENCE BOOKS FOR FOOD ALLERGY MANAGEMENT

- Young, Michael, C. M.D. **The Peanut Allergy Answer Book,** *Second Edition,* Fair Winds Press, Gloucester, MA. 2006.
  A comprehensive overview of peanut allergy.

- Sicherer Scott H. M.D. **Understanding *and* Managing Your Child's Food Allergies**, The John Hopkins University Press, Baltimore, Maryland, 2006
  Thoughtful and thorough guide to food allergies and their management.

- Sicherer, Scott H. M.D. **The Complete Peanut Allergy Handbook**, Berkley Books, N.Y., N.Y. 2005.
  Information about peanut allergies in a question and answer format.

- Hannaway, Paul J. **On the Nature of Food Allergy**, Lighthouse Press, Marblehead, MA 2007
  Information on a variety of subjects related to food allergies explained in an easy-to-read style.

- **The School Nurse's Source Book of Individualized Healthcare Plans**, Arnold, Martha J. and Silkworth, Cynthia K., Editors, Sunrise River Press, North Branch, MN, 1999.
  Comprehensive information on useful applications for individualized healthcare plans, including individualized healthcare plans with 504 Plans.

- Collins, Lisa Cipriano, M.A., M.F.T. **Caring For Your Child With Severe Food Allergies** John Wiley & Sons, Inc., N.Y. 2000.
  Helpful advice for families and caregivers of children with severe food allergies.

- Barber, Marianne S. **The Parent's Guide to Food Allergies** Henry Holt and Company, an Owl Book, N.Y. 2001.
  Clear and complete advice from the experts on raising a food-allergic child.

- Coss, Linda Marienhoff **How To Manage Your Child's Life-Threatening Food Allergies** Plumtree Press, Lake, Forest, CA. 2004.
  Practical tips for everyday life.

- Herbst, Sharon Tyler **The New Food Lover's Companion** Barron's Educational Series, Hauppauge, N.Y. Third edition 2001.
  Comprehensive definitions of nearly 6000 food, drink, and culinary terms.

- Igoe, Robert S. Hui, Y.H. **Dictionary of Food Ingredients** Fourth Edition, Aspen Publisher, Inc., Gaithersburg, Maryland 2001.
  A great source of information on over 1,000 food ingredients.

- Zukin, Jane **Dairy-Free Cookbook** Prima Health, Lava Ridge Court, Roseville, CA. 1998.
  Information on milk allergy and lactose intolerance; includes dairy-free recipes.

- Aldrich, Patricia, M.S. **Mommy's Best Recipes** G & R Publishing Company, Waverly, IA. 2001.
  Fun recipes that are dairy, soy, peanut and tree nut free.

- Coss, Linda Marienhoff **What's To Eat?** Plumtree Press, Lake Forest, CA 2000.
  The milk-free, egg-free, nut-free food allergy cookbook.

- Kidder, Beth **The Milk-Free Kitchen** Henry Holt and Company, N.Y. 1991.
  Living well without dairy products.

- Taylor, Steve, Ph.D., and Munoz-Furlong, Anne **Understanding Food Labels** The Food Allergy And Anaphylaxis Network, Fairfax, VA. 1999.
  A great reference to aid in understanding food labels.

- **Grocery Manufacturers Directory** The Food Allergy and Anaphylaxis Network, Fairfax, VA. 1999.
  Phone numbers and website addresses for the world's best known brands of foods.

REFERENCE LIST OF BOOKS & VIDEOS FOR CHILDREN

Videos available from the *Food Allergy and Anaphylaxis Network*, www.foodallergy.org:

- Video**:** **"Alexander, The Elephant Who Couldn't Eat Peanuts"** *Preschool through early elementary age. Discussion guide also available.*

- Video**:** **"Friends Helping Friends: Make It Your Goal!"** *Middle school age.*

Video available from www.pbskids.org:

- Video: **"Binky Goes Nuts"** an **Arthur** video. *Preschool and early elementary age.*

Books available from the *Food Allergy and Anaphylaxis Network*, www.foodallergy.org.

- **Alexander** **Book Series** *Preschool and Elementary Age*

  Alexander and His Pals Visit The Main Street School

  Alexander's Special Holiday Treat

  Alexander Goes Out to Eat

  Alexander Goes To a Birthday Party

  Alexander Goes Trick Or Treating

  Alexander's First Plane Ride

  Alexander's Special Holiday Treat

Alexander's First Babysitter

Alexander the Elephant Who Couldn't Eat Peanuts Coloring Book

A Special Day At School

Always Be Prepared

- **Anthony Goes To a Restaurant** *Upper Elementary and Middle School Age.*

- **How Lenny Found Out About His Food Allergy** *Elementary Age.*

- **Kim Learns How To Take Care of Herself** *Elementary Age.*

- **Kim Goes To Camp** *Elementary Age.*

- **Learning To Live With Food Allergies: Tips For Parents and Teens** Pamphlet.

- **Let's Party: Themes, Tips, and Recipes** *Elementary Age.*

- **Susie's Sister Has a Food Allergy** *Elementary Age.*

- **Stories From the Heart : A Collection of Essays From Teens With Food Allergies** Volume I and Volume II.

- Clowes, Gina **One of the Gang** AuthorHouse, Bloomington, Indiana 2009.
  A picture-themed book for young children which encourages discussion about food allergies, feelings and coping.

- Heather Mehra and Kerry McNamara, Co-Creators **"No Biggie Bunch" Book Series** www.nobiggiebunch.com. *Preschool and Elementary Age.*

Everyday Cool with Food Allergies

Dairy-Free Dino-Licious Dig

Trade-or-Treat Halloween

Peanut-Free Tea for Three

Sports-tastic Birthday Party Book

- Nassau, Elizabeth Sussman **The Peanut Butter Jam** Health Press, Santa Fe, NM 2001. *Pre-school and early elementary age. A child's reaction to having food allergies.*

- Rogers, Robyn **No Lobster, Please!** Heartstone Publishing, P.O. Box 129, Norfolk, MA 2003. *Elementary Age.* (Available through FAAN).

- Smith, Nicole Cody, **The Allergic Cow** Jungle Communications Inc., 2004. *Preschool-2nd Grade.*

- Ureel, Jessica **The Peanut Pickle** First Page Publications, 12103 Merriman, Livonia, MI 2004. www.peanutallergykids.com. *Elementary Age.*

- Weiner, Ellen **Taking Food Allergies To School** JayJo Books. LLC., P.O. Box 213, Valley Park, MO 1999 www.jayjo.com. *Elementary Age.*

LIST OF RESOURCES

American Academy of Allergy, Asthma & Immunology
555 East Wells Street, Suite 1100
Milwaukee, WI 53202
Ph: 414-272-6071
www.aaaai.org

American Academy of Pediatrics
141 Northwest Point Blvd.
Elk Grove Village, IL. 60007
Ph: 847-434-4000
www.aap.org

American College of Allergy, Asthma & Immunology
85 W. Algonquin Road, Suite 550
Arlington Heights, IL 60005
Ph: 847-427-1200
www.acaai.org

Asthma & Allergy Foundation of America (AAFA)
8201 Corporate Drive
Suite 1000
Landover, Maryland 20785
Ph: 800-727-8462
www.aafa.org
(Check for regional offices)

Centers for Disease Control and Prevention
Division of Adolescent and School Health
4770 Buford Highway, NE
MS K29
Atlanta, Georgia, 30341
Ph: 800-232-4636
www.cdc.gov

Dey Pharmaceutical Company
P.O. Box 4954
Trenton, N.J. 08650
www.dey.com

Educating For Food Allergies, LLC (EFFA)
Contacts: Jan Hanson, M.A.
80 Washington Street, Building 0-53
Norwell, MA 02061
Ph: 781-982-7029 Fax: 781-982-7037
Email: foodallergyed@verizon.net
www.foodallergyed.com

The Food Allergy & Anaphylaxis Network (FAAN)
11781 Lee Jackson Highway, Suite 160
Fairfax, VA 22033
Ph: 800-929-4040
www.foodallergy.org

Food Allergy Initiative (FAI)
515 Madison Avenue, Suite 1912
N.Y.C., N.Y. 10022-5403
Ph: 855-324-9604
www.FoodAllergyInitiative.org

Food and Nutrition Information Center
National Agricultural Library/USDA
10301 Baltimore Ave., Room 304
Beltsville, MD 20705-2351
www.nal.usda.gov

Massachusetts Dept. of Education
350 Main Street
Malden, MA 02148
Ph: 781-338-3000
www.doe.mass.edu

Massachusetts Dept. of Public Health
250 Washington Street
Boston, MA 02108-4619
Ph: 617-624-5470
www.mass.gov/DPH

National Association of School Nurses, Inc.
8484 Georgia Avenue
Suite 420
Silver Spring, MD 20910
Ph: 240-821-1130
www.nasn.org

The National Institute of Allergy and Infectious Diseases
Office of Communications and Government Relations
6610 Rockledge Drive, MSC 6612
Bethesda, MD 20892
Ph: 866-284-4107
www.niaid.nih.gov

Shionogi Pharma, Inc.
5 Concourse Pkwy
Suite 1800
Atlanta, Georgia, 30328
Ph: 800-461-3696 (Twinject)
Ph: 800-849-9707 (Adrenaclick)
www.shionogi.com

USDA Food and Nutrition Service
3101 Park Center Drive
Alexandria, VA 22302
Ph: 703-305-2062
www.fns.usda.gov/cnd/guidance

U.S. Department of Education
Office for Civil Rights
Customer Service Team
400 Maryland Avenue, SW
Washington, D.C. 20202-1100
Ph: 800-421-3481
Email: OCR.@ed.gov www2.ed.gov/ocr

ABOUT THE AUTHOR

Jan Hanson conducted her first educational workshop on the management of food allergies to school personnel in 1996. As she continued with this work, she founded the consulting company, *Educating For Food Allergies, LLC* (EFFA) in 2001, in order to further assist school staff and families in their efforts to develop effective and reasonable procedures meant to keep children with food allergies safe and fully engaged in their school programs. Her focus also includes helping to ensure that protocols are in place which address the emotional and social needs of these students. She has assisted in the development and writing of school district policy on life-threatening food allergies, and co-authored *"A Recipe for Managing Life-Threatening Food Allergies at School"* published by *Asthma Magazine* in 2002. She was a speaker at the 10th Annual Food Safety Conference hosted by the University of Rhode Island, and is a frequent speaker at informational support group meetings sponsored by the Asthma and Allergy Foundation of America, New England Chapter. Her expertise and practical approach have benefited teachers and school administrators, as well as families who seek guidance on this issue throughout New England. To date, over 250 Massachusetts school nurses have attended her workshops. Her consulting company is registered with the Massachusetts Department of Education to provide professional development points for teachers who attend her programs, and also meets the qualifications of the Massachusetts Board of Registration in Nursing to provide contact hours towards continuing education for nurses who complete her workshops. She is a professional member of the Massachusetts School Nurse Organization and the National Association of School Nurses. Ms. Hanson has her B.A. in Psychology from Mount Holyoke College and her M.A. in Higher Education Administration from Boston College. She has a son who was diagnosed at the age of 15 months with multiple life threatening food allergies and another son who was diagnosed with a walnut allergy at 18 years of age.

Jan Hanson's comprehensive, thorough and detailed handbook is an extraordinarily valuable tool for parents of children with food allergies and the educators who must keep these students safe and ready to learn. She offers clear and practical advice that will help families and schools to be successful partners in meeting the needs of children with food allergies. Hanson has been a popular speaker at our educational support groups over the past decade, and our members have benefitted tremendously from her expertise. This book is an important way to make her immense knowledge available to a much wider audience.

Sharon Schumack
Director of Education Programs
Asthma & Allergy Foundation of America, New England Chapter